Handbook of
ICU PROTOCOLS

Handbook of
ICU PROTOCOLS

Author

Shaila Shodhan Kamat
MBBS DA MD (Anesthesiology)
(Retd.) Professor and Head
Department of Anesthesiology
Goa Medical College
Bambolim, Goa, India

Co-author

Nimisha Parkar
MD DNB (Anesthesiology) IDCCM
Associate Consultant Intensivist
Intensive Care Unit
Manipal Hospitals
Panaji, Goa, India

Foreword

Muralidhar K

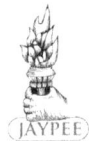

JAYPEE BROTHERS MEDICAL PUBLISHERS
The Health Sciences Publisher
New Delhi | London

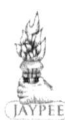

Jaypee Brothers Medical Publishers (P) Ltd.

Headquarters

Jaypee Brothers Medical Publishers (P) Ltd
EMCA House, 23/23-B
Ansari Road, Daryaganj
New Delhi 110 002, India
Landline: +91-11-23272143, +91-11-23272703
+91-11-23282021, +91-11-23245672
Email: jaypee@jaypeebrothers.com

Corporate Office

Jaypee Brothers Medical Publishers (P) Ltd
4838/24, Ansari Road, Daryaganj
New Delhi 110 002, India
Phone: +91-11-43574357
Fax: +91-11-43574314
Email: jaypee@jaypeebrothers.com

Overseas Office

JP Medical Ltd.
83, Victoria Street, London
SW1H 0HW (UK)
Phone: +44 20 3170 8910
Fax: +44 (0)20 3008 6180
Email: info@jpmedpub.com

Website: www.jaypeebrothers.com
Website: www.jaypeedigital.com

© 2024, Jaypee Brothers Medical Publishers

The views and opinions expressed in this book are solely those of the original contributor(s)/author(s) and do not necessarily represent those of editor(s) or publisher of the book.

All rights reserved. No part of this publication may be reproduced, stored or transmitted in any form or by any means, electronic, mechanical, photo copying, recording or otherwise, without the prior permission in writing of the publishers.

All brand names and product names used in this book are trade names, service marks, trademarks or registered trademarks of their respective owners. The publisher is not associated with any product or vendor mentioned in this book.

Medical knowledge and practice change constantly. This book is designed to provide accurate, authoritative information about the subject matter in question. However, readers are advised to check the most current information available on procedures included and check information from the manufacturer of each product to be administered, to verify the recommended dose, formula, method and duration of administration, adverse effects and contra indications. It is the responsibility of the practitioner to take all appropriate safety precautions. Neither the publisher nor the author(s)/editor(s) assume any liability for any injury and/or damage to persons or property arising from or related to use of material in this book.

This book is sold on the understanding that the publisher is not engaged in providing professional medical services. If such advice or services are required, the services of a competent medical professional should be sought.

Every effort has been made where necessary to contact holders of copyright to obtain permission to reproduce copyright material. If any have been inadvertently overlooked, the publisher will be pleased to make the necessary arrangements at the first opportunity.

Inquiries for bulk sales may be solicited at: jaypee@jaypeebrothers.com

Handbook of ICU Protocols

First Edition: **2024**

ISBN: 978-93-5696-395-5

Dedicated to

*My **loving brother, Mr Pradeep Vassudev Naik**
who has always supported to me*

*My **loving friends, Dr Bharati Anil Sardessai** and
Dr Beena Alhad Kantak for their
unconditional love, guidance, and **support***

*My **dear friend** and **classmate**,
Dr Antonio Rodrigues who looked after
my mother like his own mother*

*My **dear housekeepers**,
**Mrs Kuste Anant Khandeparker and
(Late) Mrs Sumati Somnath Hadphadkar**
because of their doting love, I could manage family
and profession happily and without stress*

*All my **patients** whose **unseen blessings**
helped me to complete this book*

Foreword

I am delighted to go through the *Handbook of ICU Protocols* written by Professor Shaila Shodhan Kamat and Nimisha Parkar, the prolific authors in the domain of anesthesiology and critical care.

Their writings are remarkably simple to understand, comprehend, and implement in a critical care scenario in either the operating rooms or critical care. Their publications are extremely popular among trainees and practicing physicians.

This handbook deals with a practical approach to intensive care unit (ICU) management and is a **valuable guide** to ICU physicians and trainees in managing critically ill patients. Its format is **user-friendly** and serves as a **quick reference manual** to aid **quick decision-making** in critical situations.

This book comprises 64 chapters grouped into 12 sections to cover various aspects of patient care in the ICU. In addition to clinical care of critically ill patients, it is **noteworthy** that this handbook includes sections on **documentation** and **administration** of the ICU.

I am convinced that this handbook will be of **immense benefit** to the intensivists and other healthcare professionals involved in the management of ICU. I would like to congratulate the authors for bringing out a valuable contribution that will be a **boon** to the intensive care personnel.

Thank you.

Muralidhar K
MD FIACTA FICA MBA FASE PhD
Director (Academic), Senior Consultant, and Professor
Department of Anesthesia and Intensive Care
Narayana Institute of Cardiac Sciences
Narayana Health City, Bengaluru
Professor, International Health
University of Minnesota, USA
Dean, Indian College of Anesthesiologists
Principal, Narayana Hrudayalaya Institute of
Allied Health Sciences
Bengaluru, Karnataka, India

Preface

When you kneel before God
He stands up for you
And when He stands up for you
No one can stand against you

We have always believed in smooth functioning of any department, better care of patients and that every department must devise protocols. This is particularly true for intensive care unit (ICU) which is the most critical area of any hospital. "How to build protocols in the system so that the hospital can provide ultimate care to patients in ICU?" is a question which has been asked, debated, and discussed a number of times.

This book is about ICU practices and guides **ICU doctors, trainees**, and **postgraduate students** in managing critically ill patients right from the **time of admission**, directs in taking daily rounds for the **patient assessment**, and serves as a **quick reference** manual to undertake bedside decisions.

It is a reader friendly handbook and comprises of **64 chapters** grouped into **12 sections** to cover various aspects of ICU practices. The aim of this book is to augment clinical teaching and inspire a more detailed study and further reading of the topics included.

It provides key points for the management of commonly encountered **conditions** or **problems** in patients admitted in ICU, including **troubleshooting** of mechanical ventilator. It also lays down salient points to remember, pertaining to **infection control** practices in ICU which are applicable to doctors and nursing staff.

Not only clinical, but also topics related to **documentation** and **administration** of the critical care unit are **highlighted**.

The book is **simple, practical,** and **basic** which is our specialty of writing. It will definitely be very useful for ICU **doctors**, ICU **technicians**, and ICU **nursing staff**. The book is intended to be useful in **day-to-day practice**.

We would be pleased and our efforts would be deemed worthwhile, if readers find the book useful as a **concise, up-to-date guide** for **day-to-day work** in an ICU setup.

Shaila Shodhan Kamat
Nimisha Parkar

Acknowledgments

Never lose your hope,
A single leaf can be a beginning of a forest.

Many of us may be fortunate to have supportive families, but very few of us are fortunate to have dedicated teachers, devoted pupils, and endearing family.

First and foremost, I want to offer this endeavor to **God** for always being my friend. I very strongly believe that God is **my friend**; he blesses me with wisdom, determination, health, and a strong support system.

I would like to express my gratitude to my sincere and hardworking student **Dr Nimisha Parkar** (now colleague) who constantly encouraged me to write this book. I take **pride to mention** that she is the Co-Author of this book.

I would also like to thank **Dr Deepa C** [ex-Lecturer, Goa Medical College (GMC)] who helped me to implement protocols in ICU during her posting in GMC. I would like to mention my special thanks to **Dr Marzook Sheikh** (Consultant Microbiologist) for helping me to implement decontamination protocols for environment and equipments in ICU.

I would also like to express my special **gratitude** to **Dr Muralidhar Kanchi**, one of the greatest anesthesiologists, for his valuable suggestions and for gracing the book by writing the foreword.

I also thank my loving daughter **Mrs Asmani Venkatram Shirgaonkar** for designing the aesthetically beautiful cover page of the book.

The book would not have been completed without the constant support of my family, extended family, friends, and well-wishers, who are too numerous to mention individually.

I am very thankful to **all my students** (present and past) whose love, inspiration, and wholehearted admiration for my teaching has always been a great strength to me for my continuous academic and spiritual growth.

Last but not the least, I am extremely thankful to Shri Jitendar P Vij (Group Chairman), Mr Ankit Vij (Managing Director), Mr MS Mani (Group President), Ms Chetna Malhotra (Senior Director—Professional Publishing, Marketing, and Business Development), Ms Pooja Bhandari (Director—Production), and Mr Akhilesh Saxena (Publishing Coordinator) of M/s Jaypee Brothers Medical Publishers (P) Ltd, New Delhi, India, for constant encouragement.

Contents

SECTION 1
Admission Protocol and Checklist

1. ICU Admission Policy 3
2. Checklist for Receiving New Patient in ICU 7
3. Investigations to be done on ICU Admission 10
4. Routine Investigations in ICU 11

SECTION 2
Daily Assessment in ICU and Infection Control

5. FAST HUGS BID 19
6. Drug Dilution for Infusions in ICU—
   Drug Name, Dose, and Concentration 21
7. Drop Rate Calculation of Fluids 24
8. Tips on Intravenous Fluids 25
9. Protocol for Bedside Infection Control Practices 27
10. Protocol for Endotracheal Suctioning 31
11. Protocols for Insertion and Handling of
    Central Venous Catheter 36
12. Protocol for Handling of Arterial Line 39
13. Protocol for Foley's Catheterization and
    Community-acquired Urinary Tract Infection Bundle 42

SECTION 3
Tracheostomy and Prevention of VAP

14. Tracheostomy in ICU 47
15. Protocol for Care of Patient with Tracheostomy Tube 51
16. Protocol for Change of Tracheostomy 52
17. Strategies in ICU to Prevent VAP 55

SECTION 4
Cardiorespiratory Arrest in ICU

18. Adult Tachycardia Algorithm Based on
    American Heart Association 2020 59
19. Adult Bradycardia Algorithm Based on
    American Heart Association 2020 60
20. Adult Cardiac Arrest Algorithm Based on
    the Guidelines by American Heart
    Association 2020 61
21. Defibrillation Usage in ICU 62

SECTION 5
Acid–Base Imbalance and Dyselectrolytemia

22. Sampling of Arterial Blood Gas 69
23. Steps of Arterial Blood Gases Interpretation 73
24. Protocol for Potassium Correction in Hypokalemia 79
25. Protocol for Treatment of Hyperkalemia 81

26. Hyponatremia Algorithm 83
27. Protocol for Sodium Correction in Hyponatremia.............86
28. Protocol to Calculate Rate of Infusion for 3% NaCl 87
29. Protocol for Hypernatremia 89

SECTION 6
General Protocols

30. Protocol for Nutrition in ICU 93
31. Protocol of Neuromonitoring in ICU...................................96
32. Protocol of Glucose Control in ICU................................... 101
33. Protocol for Bedsore Prevention and Care 106
34. Protocol for Antibiotic Usage in ICU 110
35. Protocol for Organ Donor Management 120

SECTION 7
Key Points in Ventilating Common ICU Admissions

36. Key Points in Ventilating Respiratory Failure.................. 131
37. Key Points in Ventilating Postoperative
    (Normal Lung) Patient.. 136
38. Key Points in Ventilating Neuromuscular Diseases 139
39. Key Points in Ventilating Head/Brain Injury.................... 146
40. Key Points in Ventilating Severe Asthma......................... 151
41. Key Points in Ventilating Chronic Obstructive
    Pulmonary Disease 155

42. Key Points in Ventilating Acute Respiratory Distress Syndrome 162

43. Key Points in Care of Patients on Long-term Mechanical Ventilator 169

44. Ventilator Troubleshooting 171

45. Weaning Criteria 175

SECTION 8
Blood Transfusion

46. Protocol for Blood Transfusion in ICU 181

47. Protocol for Massive Blood Transfusion 187

SECTION 9
Scoring System in ICU

48. SOFA Score 191

49. Child Pugh Score for Liver Disease 193

50. Clinical Pulmonary Infection Score for Ventilator Associated Pneumonia 194

51. Wells Score for Predicting Risk of Pulmonary Embolism (PE) 195

52. Pulmonary Embolism Severity Index (PESI) Score 196

53. Acute Physiological and Chronic Health Evaluation (APACHE)-II Score 197

54. Score for Atrial Fibrillation Stroke Risk, CHA_2DS_2VASc 199

SECTION 10
Bedside Hemodialysis in ICU

55. Protocol for Dialysis 203

SECTION 11
Documentation and Checklists

56. Protocol for Intubation Trolley 209
57. Protocol for Making Sterile Sets 211
58. Transfer Out/Death Report 212
59. Protocol to Write Death Report 214

SECTION 12
Waste Management and Decontamination

60. Anesthetic Assistant or Technician: Decontamination of Environment and Equipments in ICU 217
61. Nursing Staff: Decontamination of Environment and Equipments in ICU 219
62. Housekeeping Personnel: Decontamination of Environment and Equipments in ICU 220
63. ICU Attendant: Decontamination of Environment and Equipments in ICU 224
64. Waste Disposal 225

Glossary 227

SECTION 1
Admission Protocol and Checklist

1. ICU Admission Policy
2. Checklist for Receiving New Patient in ICU
3. Investigations to be done on ICU Admission
4. Routine Investigations in ICU

CHAPTER 1: ICU Admission Policy

Admission in intensive care unit (ICU) involves utilization of limited and valuable resources in critically ill individuals, rigorous medical, and nursing attention with highly specialized therapeutic and monitoring equipments. It is multidisciplinary specialty providing comprehensive diagnostic and therapeutic services for patients, and should be reserved and prioritized for patients suffering from **potentially recoverable and reversible** diseases who can benefits from more **detailed observation** and treatment than is generally available in standard wards and departments.

Although such criteria cannot be strictly delineated, the following form the basis of defining institutional ICU admission policy:

1. Acute failure of two or more organ systems
2. Isolated acute respiratory failure or respiratory support for >12 hours
3. Single acute organ system failure (OSF) with one or more chronic OSFs

High-dependency care is an intermediate level of care provided for patients with, or at risk of:
1. A single acute organ system failure (OSF) excluding respiratory failure
2. Chronic stable failure of two organ systems
3. Chronic unstable failure of a single organ system

Patient selection for critical care services can also be facilitated by analyzing the likelihood of benefit in terms of **survival. Likely outcome** is a major consideration, on the basis of which, patients can be categorized into one of the following four groups:
1. Expected to survive or potentially recoverable
2. Prognosis uncertain
3. Death probable shortly whatever is done
4. Death apparently imminent

It is suggested that intensive care is considered for the **first two categories** of patients. Patient whose death is probable in spite of active intervention should form the basis of detailed discussion and counseling, at the highest clinical level, with regard to any perceived benefit which is likely to accrue.

Any one of the following qualifies a patient requiring critical care services:
- Patient requiring ventilator support including noninvasive ventilation (NIV), high-flow nasal oxygen
- Patient requiring basic and advanced hemodynamic monitoring and support, needing vasopressors, inotropes, intra-aortic balloon pump

- Patient who requires renal replacement therapy [Continuous renal replacement therapy (**CRRT**), sustained low-efficiency dialysis (**SLED**)], who are unstable hemodynamically.
- Severe sepsis with or without shock
- Patient admitted to ICU for monitoring of neurological status, e.g., all acute strokes, subarachnoid hemorrhage (**SAH**), status epilepticus, altered sensorium (who would require airway protection), traumatic brain injury if Glasgow Coma Scale (GCS) is **<8–10**, and seizure disorder.
- All victims of major trauma with hemodynamic instability, chest, and abdominal trauma. Any patient with active bleeding needing frequent monitoring of hemoglobin and coagulation status
- Requirement of more than one drug infusions
- Following major surgeries for monitoring of postoperative complications
- Patients needing **NIV** beyond 48 hours after extubation
- Patients having acute kidney injury (**AKI**) on chronic kidney injury (**CKD**)
- Upper gastrointestinal (**UGI**) bleed with or without shock
- All poisoning for first 48 hours

EXCLUSION CRITERIA

The following categories of patients are generally considered **unsuitable** for admission to the ICU:

1. Patients with disseminated malignancy

2. Patients with terminal organ failure following the natural progression of a chronic condition:
   - Terminal respiratory failure in chronic bronchitis
   - Chronic respiratory failure secondary to progressive neuromuscular disorders
3. Patients requiring minimal monitoring, admission requested due to ward staff shortages
4. Patients more appropriately referred to a specialist unit

These broad criteria aid in efficient utilization of ICU facilities and services, however, it is finally the **clinician's assessment** and judgment on case-to-case basis to decide regarding ICU admission.

CHAPTER 2: Checklist for Receiving New Patient in ICU

BEFORE RECEIVING THE PATIENT

- Vacant intensive care unit (ICU) bed has to be kept ready.
- Cardiac monitor to be ready with modules.
- Ambu bag with tubing and reservoir, transducer, electrocardiogram (ECG) cable, and intravenous (IV) stand
- Patient trolley with stethoscope and torch
- Ventilator to be checked (O_2 connection, working condition, and alarms)
- Transducer to be ready if patient is having central venous line (CVC) and arterial line
- Suction to be checked (connection and working condition)
- Intubation trolley
- Arterial blood gas (ABG) syringes and emergency drugs, head pillow to be ready.

AFTER RECEIVING THE PATIENT

- **Receiving time** to be noted
- Wash hands before touching the patient

- Settle the patient—elevate the head end to **45°**, cover the patient, and keep warm. Provide most comfortable position
- Remove and handover **valuables** to attendants and take signature
- Catheterization of bladder, if indicated
- **Inform the relatives;** explain the patient's condition on their visit. Local contact number to be noted in the main chart
- Check the **identity band** and **admission report** of the patient
- To check vital signs, record, and inform them
- Carry out doctors' orders and send investigations, accordingly, inform references if any
- To record nursing observations, enter admission in register/computer
- Orientation to be given to patient and patient attendant

Hemodynamic parameters to be noted and charted every **30 minutes** for **4 hours** and then **hourly**.

- In postoperative patients, check drainage every **15 minutes** for **2 hours**, every **30 minutes** for **2 hours** and then hourly
- Report any **changes in hemodynamics** and **drainage** to duty intensivist and resident doctor immediately
- **Milk the drainage tubes** every **half an hourly** for **4 hours** and then **hourly** (if not contraindicated)

- Check all the ongoing infusions (concentrations, labels). Drug calculations arc to be **cross checked** by two nurses.
- Check for **oozing** from dressing site/CVC site/arterial line site. If the site is soaked, change it using sterile technique.
- Check **patient's back** immediately after arrival (if patient is stable). Report if there is any redness/hardness/skin peeling on the back, to senior in charge, and mention it in the chart
- Give **back care** every **2 hourly** for ventilator patients and **6 hourly** for extubated patients (if patient is stable)
- Dispose the waste properly
- **Enter consumables** properly and give hand over/take over in each shift with staff's signature.

All the formalities can be performed later on if patient's clinical condition warrants immediate measures

- Start oxygen, secure IV line if not already present
- Monitor heart rate, blood pressure, oxygen saturation, respiration, temperature, and sensorium
- Call emergency help if needed, crash cart to be wheeled in.

CHAPTER 3: Investigations to be done on ICU Admission

Postoperative patients	Medical patients
Hemoglobin, PCV	Hb, PCV, TC, and DC
ECG	If needed
Platelet count	Platelet count
aPTT, PT, and INR	aPTT, PT, and INR
RBSL, ABG, CXR	RBSL, ABG, and CXR
RFTs, LFTs including serum albumin	RFTs, LFTs including serum albumin
Serum Na^+, K^+, Cl^-, Ca^{2+}, Mg^{2+}	Serum electrolytes Na^+, K^+, Cl^-, Ca^2, Mg^{2+}
	Endotracheal aspirate Gram stain and culture, blood culture, urine routine/microscopy and culture as indicated

CHAPTER 4: Routine Investigations in ICU

Daily

1.	CBC	Hb, TC, DC, platelet count, and PCV
2.	RFT's	Blood urea, serum creatinine, Na^+, K^+, and Cl^-
3.		ABG
4.		RBSL

Every 72 Hours or Earlier if Needed

1.	LFTs	SGOT/PT, ALP, total protein, A:G ratio, serum bilirubin (total and direct)
2.		Serum Ca, serum Mg
3.		Serum phosphate
4.		Chest X-ray

As per Indication

1.	Bactec culture sensitivity	1.	Urine Na^+
2.	Arterial ammonia levels	2.	Serum osmolality
3.	aPTT, PT, and INR	3.	Plasma ketones (urine ketones)
4.	CH with ESR	4.	Urine sodium
5.	Gram stain	5.	Urine osmolality
6.	TFTs—T_3, T_4, TSH, free T_3, and free T_4	6.	Serum cholinesterase levels

Contd…

Contd…

7.	D-dimer	7.	AFB	Stain
8.	FDP			Culture
9.	Serum fibrinogen	8.	Serum cortisol levels	
10.	Urine for toxicology screening	9.	Cardiac enzymes	CPK-MB
11.	Hepatitis A, B, C workup			Troponin
12.	ELISA	10.	Kits	HIV
13.	Procalcitonin			Hepatitis B
14.	*Clostridium difficile* toxin assay	11.	Serum amylase	
15.	Dengue NS1 Ag	12.	Serum lipase	
16.	Falcivax	13.	Urine amylase	
17.	SMP	14.	24-hour urine protein	
18.	TB-PCR	15.	IgM Leptospira	
19.	HSV-PCR	16.	IgM dengue	

Pleural Fluid Studies and CSF Studies

1.	Biochemistry	Sugar, protein, chloride, ADA, and albumin
2.	Cytology	Malignant cells
3.	Cells counts	WBCs and RBCs
4.	Culture and sensitivity	Bacterial/fungal

1.	Chest X-ray	1.	CTPA
2.	USG	2.	ECG
3.	CT scan and HRCT	3.	2D echocardiography
		4.	EEG

Investigations Needed Based on Medical History

Preoperative diagnosis	ECG	Chest X-ray	Hct/Hb	CBC	Electrolytes	Creatinine	Glucose	Coagulation	LFTs	Drug levels	Ca
Cardiac disease											
History of myocardial infarction	X			X	±						
Chronic stable angina	X			X	±						
Congestive heart failure (CHF)	X	±									
Hypertension (HTN)	X	±			If patient is taking **Diuretics**	X					
Chronic atrial fibrillation	X									If patient is taking **Digoxin**	
Peripheral arterial disease (PAD)	X										
Valvular heart disease	X	±									

Contd...

Contd...

Preoperative diagnosis	ECG	Chest X-ray	Hct/Hb	CBC	Electrolytes	Creatinine	Glucose	Coagulation	LFTs	Drug levels	Ca
Pulmonary disease											
COPD	X	±		X	Pulmonary function tests (**PFTs**) only if symptomatic; otherwise, no tests required						
Asthma	X	±		X						If patient is taking **Theophylline**	
Liver disease											
Infectious hepatitis								X	X		
Alcohol or drug-induced hepatitis								X	X		
Tumor infiltration								X	X		
CNS disorders											
Stroke	X			X	X		X				
Seizures	X			X	X		X			X	
Diabetes	X				±	X	X			X	
Renal disease			X		X	X					
Hematologic disorders				X							

Contd...

Contd...

Preoperative diagnosis	ECG	Chest X-ray	Hct/Hb	CBC	Electrolytes	Creatinine	Glucose	Coagulation	LFTs	Drug levels	Ca
Coagulopathies				x				x			
Tumor	x			x							
Vascular disorders or aneurysms	x		x								
Malignant disease				x							
Endocrine disorders											
Hyperthyroidism	x		x		x	Thyroid function test					x
Hypothyroidism	x		x		x						
Cushing disease				x	x		x				
Addison disease				x	x		x				
Hyperparathyroidism	x		x		x						x
Hypoparathyroidism	x				x						x
Morbid obesity	x	±					x				
Malabsorption or poor nutrition	x			x	x	x	x				

Contd...

Contd...

Preoperative diagnosis	ECG	Chest X-ray	Hct/Hb	CBC	Electrolytes	Creatinine	Glucose	Coagulation	LFTs	Drug levels	Ca
Select drug therapies											
Digoxin (digitalis)	X				±					X	
Anticoagulants			X					X			
Phenytoin										X	
Phenobarbital										X	
Diuretics					X	X					
Corticosteroids				X			X				
Chemotherapy				X		±					
Aspirin or NSAIDs											
Theophylline										X	

(COPD: chronic obstructive pulmonary disease; CBC: complete blood count; Hct: hematocrit; LFTs: liver function tests; NSAIDs: nonsteroidal anti-inflammatory drugs)

X - Investigation to be done   **±** - **Advisable**

SECTION 2

Daily Assessment in ICU and Infection Control

5. FAST HUGS BID
6. Drug Dilution for Infusions in ICU—Drug Name, Dose, and Concentration
7. Drop Rate Calculation of Fluids
8. Tips on Intravenous Fluids
9. Protocol for Bedside Infection Control Practices
10. Protocol for Endotracheal Suctioning
11. Protocols for Insertion and Handling of Central Venous Catheter
12. Protocol for Handling of Arterial Line
13. Protocol for Foley's Catheterization and Community-acquired Urinary Tract Infection Bundle

CHAPTER 5

FAST HUGS BID

Give Your Patient FAST HUG (at least) Once a Day

F Feed	**Route:** Enteral, parenteral or nil by mouth	Intravenous (IV) metoclopramide **10** mg **8** hourly may be added
A Analgesia	Assess Visual Analog Scale (**VAS**) pain score	**500** µg fentanyl + **25** mg midazolam in **50** mL NS @ **2–6** mL/h **Stop** infusion at **5 AM** to assess the patient; restart if required
S Sedation	Glasgow Coma Scale (**GCS**) and sedation scores Richmond Agitation and Sedation Score (**RASS**)	
T Thromboprophylaxis	Pharmacological or mechanical sequential compression device	**Enoxaparin 0.4 mL** subcutaneous once a day, **Dalteparin** (Fragmin) **5,000 U** subcutaneous once a day
H Head-end elevation	30–45°	
U Ulcer prophylaxis	**Ranitidine:** 50 mg IV twice a day	**Pantoprazole:** **40** mg IV once a day

Contd…

Contd...

G **Glycemic control**	To maintain glycemic control	**140–180** mg/dL, IV infusion of regular insulin, **1–2 hourly** random blood sugar level (RBSL) monitoring
S **Spontaneous breathing trial**	**Weaning mode:** Pressure support **(PS)**/continuous positive airway pressure **(CPAP), T-piece**	
B **Bowel movements**	Indication of laxative, enema. Presence of ileus and gastroparesis	
I **Indwelling catheter**	Days since insertion of invasive lines and tubes, assessment for possibility of infection, requirement, **plan for removal**	
D **Drug de-escalation**	Daily assessment for possibility of **antibiotic de-escalation**	

CHAPTER 6

Drug Dilution for Infusions in ICU—Drug Name, Dose, and Concentration

$$\frac{\mu g/kg/min \times \textbf{body weight (kg)} \times 60}{\textbf{Concentration (}\mu g/mL\textbf{)}} = mL/h$$

$$\frac{mL \times \textbf{Concentration (}\mu g/mL\textbf{)}}{\textbf{Body weight (kg)} \times 60} = \mu g/kg/min$$

Drug name	Dose	Concentration	Volume	Fluid for dilution	Dilution
Adrenaline	0.05–0.1 µg/kg/min	2 mg	50 mL	Normal saline	40 µg/mL
Noradrenaline	0.05–1.0 µg/kg/min	4 mg	50 mL	Normal saline	80 µg/mL
Isoprenaline	0.05–1.5 µg/kg/min	2 mg	50 mL	Normal saline	40 µg/mL
Phenylephrine	0.5–1.0 µg/kg/min	10 mg	50 mL	Normal saline	200 µg/mL
Dopamine	2–20 µg/kg/min	200 mg	50 mL	Normal saline	4 mg/mL
Dobutamine	2–20 µg/kg/min	250 mg	50 mL	Normal saline	5 mg/mL
Vasopressin	0.01–0.04 U/min	20 U	50 mL	Normal saline	0.4 U/mL
Milrinone	2–5 µg/kg/min	10 mg	50 mL	Normal saline	200 µg/mL
Levosimendan	0.2–0.7 µg/kg/min	12.5 mg	50 mL	Normal saline	250 µg/mL

Contd...

Contd...

Drug name	Dose	Concentration	Volume	Fluid for dilution	Dilution
Amiodarone	5 mg/kg over 1 hour **(loading dose)**	300 mg	50 mL	Normal saline	6 mg/mL
	5 µg/kg/min over 23 hours	900 mg	50 mL	Normal saline	18 mg/mL
MgSO$_4$	1–2 g/h	2 g	50 mL	Normal saline	40 mg/mL
Nitroglycerin (NTG)	0.3–5 µg/kg/min	50 mg	50 mL	Normal saline	1 mg/mL
Sodium nitroprusside	0.3–10 µg/kg/min	50 mg	50 mL	Normal saline	1 mg/mL
Labetalol	0.2–2 mg/kg/h	100 mg	50 ml	Normal Saline	2 mg/mL
Pantoprazole	0.15–2.0 mg/kg/h	200 mg	50 mL	Normal saline	4 mg/mL
Esomeprazole	0.15–2.0 mg/kg/h	200 mg	50 mL	Normal saline	4 mg/mL
Fentanyl	1–2 µg/kg/h	500 µg	50 mL	Normal saline	10 µg/mL
Midazolam	0.1–0.4 mg/kg/h	25 mg	50 mL	Normal saline	0.5 mg/mL
Dexmedetomidine	1 µg/kg over 10 minutes **(loading dose)**				
	0.2–0.7 µg/kg/h	100 µg	50 mL	Normal saline	2 µg/mL
Propofol	25–100 µg/kg/min	500 µg	50 mL	–	10 mg/mL

Contd...

Contd...

Drug name	Dose	Concentration	Volume	Fluid for dilution	Dilution
Insulin	0.1 U/kg/h, then adjust according to random blood sugar level **(RBSL)**	40 U	40 mL	Normal saline	1 U/mL
Lasix (Furosemide)	0.1–0.4 mg/kg/h	200 mg	20 mL	Normal saline	10 mg/mL
Heparin	50–100 U/kg loading dose 10–25 U/kg/h according to activated partial thromboplastin clotting time **(APTT)**	25,000 U	25 mL	Normal saline	1000/mL

CHAPTER 7

Drop Rate Calculation of Fluids

For drop rate calculation for **24 hours**

Rule of Ten—Drop rate/min

Volume in **L/24 h × 10**

For drop rate calculation for **1 hour**

Rule of Four—Drop rate/min

$$\frac{\text{Volume in mL/h}}{4}$$

Routine intravenous (IV) sets

12–15 drops/min = **1 mL**

Microdrip sets—60 drops/min = **1 mL**

Number of **microdrops**/min = **Volume in mL/h**

CHAPTER 8

Tips on Intravenous Fluids

Sodium Concentration of Intravenous (IV) Fluids

IV fluid	Ringer's lactate	Isolyte P	DNS/NS	3% NaCl
Na mEq/L	130	25	154	513

Potassium Concentration of IV Fluids

IV fluid	Ringer's lactate	Isolyte P	Plasmalyte, Kabilyte
K mEq/L	4	20	5

Characteristics of IV fluids

Type of fluid	Characteristics
Most physiological	Ringer's lactate
Rich in potassium	Ringer's lactate
Avoid in liver failure	Ringer's lactate
Glucose free	Ringer's lactate Normal saline
Corrects acidosis	Ringer's lactate Isolyte P

Choice of IV fluids

Ideal initial fluid	Clinical disorders
Ringer's lactate	Burns
Ringer's lactate	Intraoperative
Ringer's lactate Normal saline	Diarrhea
Normal saline Ringer's lactate	Hypokalemic shock
Isolyte P 0.45 DNS Ringer's lactate	Pediatric maintenance

Contd...

Contd...

Characteristics of IV fluids		Choice of IV fluids	
Type of fluid	Characteristics	Ideal initial fluid	Clinical disorders
Cautious in renal failure	Ringer's lactate Isolyte P		
Isotonic	Normal saline	Normal saline	Vomiting
Rich in sodium	Normal saline Dextrose saline	Normal saline	Diabetic ketoacidosis
Rich in chloride	Normal saline, DNS		
Potassium free	Normal saline, DNS, Dextrose fluids	Normal saline avoid glucose	Stroke Neurosurgery patient
Sodium free	Dextrose solution	Dextrose solution	Starvation deficit

CHAPTER 9

Protocol for Bedside Infection Control Practices

Strict handwashing practice to be implemented, starting from the **time of entry** in the critical care unit. Handrub solution should be placed easily accessible on each bed.

Apply **handrub prior** to first patient contact.

Handwashing rather than handrub use is recommended before any sterile procedure, handling of vascular access or tracheostomy tube.

Single use **disposable oxygen masks** and **nasal prongs** should be used for each new patient.

Articles present at bedside, one per bed, namely stethoscope, thermometer, and Ambu should be cleaned after each use.

Avoid reusing disposable articles.

Handwashing and use of gloves are important protective measures to prevent the transmission of the infective agents to other susceptible patients or staff.

HANDWASHING

Moments of Handwashing

Moment **1**: Before touching a patient
Moment **2**: Before a procedure

Moment **3**: After a procedure or body fluid exposure risk
Moment **4**: After touching a patient
Moment **5**: After touching a patient's surroundings.

The minimum time for a hand scrub should be **2 minutes** before starting any procedure. Between patients a **30-second** scrub is sufficient if the patient is not grossly contaminated. A **60-second** scrub is advised after attending to a grossly contaminated patient.

Hands should be washed always after removing gloves and also before sterile gloves are worn.

Seven steps of Handwash/Handrub:
1. Palm to palm
2. Palm to back, fingers over laced
3. Palm to back, fingers inter laced
4. Fingers interlocked
5. Rotational rubbing of thumb in palm
6. Rotational rubbing of fingertips in palm
7. Rubbing of wrist

Gloves: Gloves should **not** be regarded as a **substitute** for handwashing.

Types of Gloves
1. **Examination gloves**, i.e., clear gloves, which are not sterile, used for procedures, which do not require sterile techniques.
2. **Sterile gloves** when strict asepsis is warranted.
3. **Heavy duty gloves:** Used by those involved in cleaning of soiled items.

If an individual has any cut or abrasions, these should be covered with a **waterproof adhesive plastic** dressing before wearing the gloves.

Masks: These should be to be worn to protect the eyes, nose, and mouth, wherever aerosols and splashes are expected.

Types of masks used by Healthcare workers

Type	Prevents	Diameter filtration capacity
1. Surgical mask	Protects from **droplet**	0.3 µm
2. N-95 mask	Filters up to **95%** of air borne particles	>5 µm

When removing a mask, care should be taken **to avoid** touching the part which has acted as the filter as hands can easily get contaminated with bacteria.

Isolation: Infection prevention and control precautions aimed at controlling and preventing the spread of infection.

TYPES OF ISOLATION

Barrier nursing is also called **source isolation**.

It is an isolation technique done with the intent of confining microorganisms within a given area, where the patient is the source of infection. This includes contact precautions, droplet precautions, and airborne infection prevention.

Reverse barrier nursing is also called **protective isolation**, where the patient being immunocompromised requires protection, i.e., neutropenic patient, post solid organ or hemopoietic stem cell transplantation, burns, Stevens–Johnson syndrome, and selected patients post chemotherapy.

1:1 Patient:Nurse Ratio

1. Keep adequate supply of facemasks and footwear covers.
2. Strict handwashing practices prior to entering the room.
3. Put a sign board "**Barrier Nursing**" on patient door.
4. **Restrict visitors** and individuals with any skin, respiratory, or other contagious disease should not enter the room.
5. Wash hands, put on mask, gown, and shoe cover prior to entry into the room, and wear gloves as and when required.
6. Closely look at all invasive lines, catheters, and IV site of all patients daily.
7. Use sterilized linen for the patient.

CHAPTER 10

Protocol for Endotracheal Suctioning

CLINICAL INDICATIONS FOR ENDOTRACHEAL TUBE SUCTION

- Desaturation
- Bradycardia
- Tachycardia
- Absent or decreased chest movement
- Visible secretions in endotracheal tube (ETT)
- Increased end-tidal carbon dioxide ($EtCO_2$)
- Irritability
- Coarse or decreased breath sounds
- Increased work of breathing
- Blood pressure fluctuations
- Recent history of large amounts of thick/tenacious secretions

EQUIPMENT

Functioning wall suction unit with suction tubing connected

Suction catheter for open suction (see Table below for appropriate sizes for adult patients)

Endotracheal tube size	Size of suction catheter (Fr)
6 – 7	10
7.5 – 8	12
8 – 8.5	14
9 – 10	16

Diameter of the catheter should be approximately **one third** the diameter of the ETT and should be of length to **extend 5 cm beyond the distal** end of the ETT.

Nonsterile gloves

Normal saline ampoule and syringe (if normal saline lavage required)

TECHNIQUE

- Strict asepsis
- Amount of negative pressure in suction should be adjusted to **100–150 mm Hg**
- Preoxygenate with 100% O_2. Fraction of inspired oxygen (FiO_2) should be decreased as soon as possible after suction is complete. **Oxygenation** and **hyperventilation** pre-/postsuction may **NOT** be routine but, may reduce the incidence of suction related hypoxemia and bradycardia.

- Insert the catheter gently until resistance is met and then withdraw the catheter **1 cm before** applying suction.
- **No suction** should be applied during insertion of the catheter.
- Suction application should be limited to **10–15 seconds**.
- While the catheter is being removed, it should be **twirled** between the thumb and index finger so that the catheter is exposed to larger surface areas.
- Perform **hyperoxygenation** and **hyperinflation** between suctioning.
- After the endotracheal suctioning is over, the catheter is **rinsed** in **sterile water** and used for oropharyngeal suctioning.
- Two persons should be involved during the endotracheal suctioning procedure.
- **Monitor** SpO_2, hemodynamic, and intracranial pressure (ICP).

RELATIVE CONTRAINDICATIONS
- Pulmonary edema.

COMPLICATIONS OF ETT SUCTION
- Hypoxemia
- Atelectasis
- Bradycardia
- Tachycardia
- Increased ETT CO_2 and transcutaneous CO_2

- Blood pressure fluctuations
- Decreased tidal volume
- Airway mucosal trauma
- ETT dislodgement
- Pneumothorax
- Pneumomediastinum
- Bacteremia
- Pneumonia
- Fluctuations in intracranial pressure and cerebral blood flow velocity

Lavage by instillation of normal saline into the ETT immediately prior to ETT suction:
- May aid in the removal of thick, tenacious secretions by thinning, loosening, and dislodging these secretions
- Makes the patient cough, which may loosen and dislodge secretions
- May lubricate the ETT
- May have detrimental effects on the patient, damages airway mucosa, and contributes to lower airway colonization

Normal saline **should not** be routinely instilled prior to ETT suction. It should only be instilled in patients who have thick, tenacious secretions. The amount of normal saline to use is **0.1–0.2 mL/kg**.

Document clearly:
- ETT suctioned
- Airway secretion amount and color
- Suction tolerance and significant events

Effectiveness of ETT suction should be assessed after the procedure by observing:
- Improvement in breath sounds on auscultation
- Removal of secretions
- Improved oxygen saturation, $EtCO_2$, heart rate, blood pressure, and respiratory rate
- Decreased work of breathing and improved chest rise

CHAPTER 11

Protocols for Insertion and Handling of Central Venous Catheter

WHILE INSERTING CENTRAL VENOUS CATHETER

Hand hygiene and barrier precautions by the operator to be maintained.

Select an optimal site of insertion.

Site to be prepared with **2% chlorhexidine** and draped.

WHILE HANDLING CENTRAL VENOUS CATHETER PORTS

Central venous line ports to be handled **only** after using **0.5% chlorhexidine** hand rub.

Clean the **hubs** of three-way cocks with **chlorhexidine** while administering drugs, connecting intravenous (IV) line, and also while collecting blood culture samples.

Ports have to be **flushed** with **normal saline**, or else the lumen gets blocked. **NO** air bubbles should be injected.

There should be **NO** blood stains or blood clots in the extension tubing's or in three-way stopcocks as this will lead to bacterial growth.

Label the syringes and lines specifying the infusions on flow

Change of infusion lines and three-way stopcocks every **72 hours**

Assess the insertion **site** for localized inflammation, pus, and change the catheter site if infection is suspected.

Paired blood culture samples to be sent [one from central venous catheter (CVC) and another from periphery] if **infection** is suspected.

Maximum interval between change of dressing:
1. Gauze dressing every **2** days
2. Transparent dressing every **7** days

The CVC line cannulation site is preferably changed **once** in **15** days or earlier if infected.

Daily assessment of the requirement of CVC based on the patient's clinical status and removal when **NO** more indicated.

USES OF PORTS OF CENTRAL VENOUS LINE

1. **Distal port** to be used for IV fluids, for administering drugs as bolus injection and for measurement of central venous pressure.
2. Second port (**middle port**) to be used for concentrated ions Mg^{2+}, Calcium, K^+, and sedation analgesia.
3. Third port (**proximal port**) to be used for inotropes/vasopressors/vasodilators—adrenaline, noradrenaline, dopamine, dobutamine, and nitroglycerine.

Use **one dedicated port** for **total parenteral nutrition**

Note: If only two ports are available; use the **second** port **(NOT THE DISTAL PORT)** for the purpose mentioned in 2 and 3.

CHAPTER 12

Protocol for Handling of Arterial Line

INSERTION

Sites

- Radial artery (most common)—Perform Allen's test prior to cannulation
- Ulnar artery
- Brachial artery
- Axillary artery
- Femoral arterial cannulation should be done by Seldinger technique
- Dorsalis pedis artery, posterior tibial, and superficial temporal artery (pediatric)

Device

- Arterial switch cannula (20 G)
- Central venous catheter (CVC) single lumen (18 G)

Technique

- Direct arterial cannulation
- Seldinger technique
- Ultrasonography (USG) guided
- Transfixation

Indications

- Invasive blood pressure monitoring for continuous and real time blood pressure monitoring
- Planned pharmacologic or mechanical cardiovascular manipulation
- Withdrawal of repeated blood samples and ABG sample
- Burns or obesity due to failed noninvasive blood pressure
- To derive diagnostic inferences from the arterial waveform
- Accurate titration of vasoactive drugs, antihypertensives in hypertensive crisis, and postcardiac arrest status
- Planned pharmacological and mechanical cardiovascular interventions
- Use of intra-aortic balloon pump
- During surgery and postoperatively with anticipated blood loss and large fluid shifts

COMPONENTS OF INVASIVE BLOOD PRESSURE MEASUREMENT SYSTEM

- Fluid filled tubing
- Intravenous fluid i.e. crystalloid
- Transducer
- Infusion/flushing system at flow rate of **1–3 mL/h (no heparin)**
- Signal processor, amplifier, and display
- Intra-arterial cannula

CANNULATION

- Operator should wear sterile gown, head cap, and mask and gloves.
- Prepare the **insertion site** with **2% chlorhexidine** and cannulation to be done under strict asepsis.
- **Transparent dressing** should be applied and the site should be inspected daily.

DAILY CHECK

- Site of cannula, intactness of dressing, check for back flow
- Tubing for clots, air bubbles, and kinking
- Tightness of all the connections should be ascertained.
- **Zeroing**, secure transducer level to phlebostatic axis, intersection of **fourth intercostals** space and the **midaxillary line**
- Maintain the **patency** of the arterial line
- **Never flush** the arterial line **without** checking for back flow. If any **blood clot** or **air bubble** noted in 10-cm extension then do **not flush**. If **resistance felt** during aspiration, do **not** flush.
- Maintain adequate pressure of **300 mm Hg** in a pressure bag to prevent backflow
- Assessment of the requirement of arterial line and early removal of arterial line when **no** more indicated and as a part of source control measures in case of sepsis.
- On **removal** of cannula apply adequate pressure and pressure bandage

Protocol for Foley's Catheterization and Community-acquired Urinary Tract Infection Bundle

CHAPTER 13

Note down
a. Date of insertion
b. **Indications for catheterization**
   - Surgery performed
   - Acute renal failure
   - On inotropes
   - Diuretic administration in high dose
   - Urinary obstruction/incontinence/retention
c. Catheterization done by

URINARY CATHETER INSERTION BUNDLE

- Perform surgical handwash prior to insertion of catheter
- Aseptic precautions to be adhered to prior to catheterization (i.e., sterile gloves and drape). **Non touch technique** as far as possible.
- Urethral meatus is to be cleaned with **normal saline** prior to catheter insertion
- Foley's catheter balloon to be filled with **sterile water**.

DAILY REVIEW

- **Assess** if urinary catheter is still required.
- Check if **closed drainage system** is maintained.

- Daily meatal and perineal care to be given.
- Drainage bag has to be kept **above floor** but **below the level of bladder**. Drainage bag should **not be raised** above the bladder height **without clamping the tube**.
- Catheter to be secured with **tape over thigh** to prevent movement.
- Urinary bag to be emptied once it is **two-thirds filled**. When emptying the urinary bag, it should be **completely** emptied to **prevent** the build-up of organisms in stagnant urine.
- See that the patient is **not lying over the catheter** or **tube causing obstruction** of urine flow.

To send sample for **urine culture** as and when indicated.

If catheter is changed:

a. Date of change
b. Reason for change

SECTION 3
Tracheostomy and Prevention of VAP

14. Tracheostomy in ICU
15. Protocol for Care of Patient with Tracheostomy Tube
16. Protocol for Change of Tracheostomy
17. Strategies in ICU to Prevent VAP

CHAPTER 14

Tracheostomy in ICU

Tracheostomy may be performed either as a surgical procedure in the operating room or as a percutaneous procedure within the intensive care setting, when artificial airway is required **longer** than **7-10** days to facilitate weaning.

Other indications are:
- Upper airway obstruction or malformation
- Repeated intubations, failed extubation
- Presence of complications of endotracheal intubation, glottic incompetence, sleep apnea, and chronic inability to clear secretions

EQUIPMENT AND REQUIREMENTS FOR TRACHEOSTOMY IN ICU

- Consent and information provided to patient and significant others
- Sterile dressing pack, gown/gloves/trolley
- Disposable dressing pack
- Percutaneous/surgical tracheostomy set
- Tracheostomy of appropriate size (fenestrated/unfenestrated)

- 1% or 2% Lignocaine with adrenaline, Lignocaine jelly
- Syringe
- Stethoscope
- Suction catheter (appropriate size)
- **End-tidal carbon dioxide ($EtCO_2$) monitor**

Pre-procedure

- Check coagulation and platelet profile.
- **Nil per oral 6 hours** prior to procedure and aspirate NG tube.
- Do a thorough **oropharyngeal suction**.
- **Deflate the cuff** of the ET tube; perform laryngoscopy and carefully withdraw the ET tube until the cuff is just visible at the vocal cords. **Note the mark** and fix the ET tube at that mark after reinflating the ET cuff.
- Check tracheostomy tube is patent, inflate the cuff and submerge under water, **check for leaks**, deflate, and cover with Lignocaine jelly.
- Ensure **$EtCO_2$** monitoring is in situ.
- Ensure all **emergency equipment** are ready and in working order.
- Ensure patient is monitored.
- Ensure **adequate sedation** as ordered.
- Position patient appropriately usually after sedation.
- **Preoxygenate** with 100% O_2 for 3–5 minutes.

During Procedure

- Assist the procedure, but always remain vigilant regarding the patient's vitals.
- **Deflate the cuff** of the ET tube and **remove the ET tube** out of larynx only after confirming the position of the tracheostomy tube using $EtCO_2$ monitoring, observation of chest rise, and auscultation of chest.
- Secure tracheostomy appropriately with tapes or soft collar.
- Connect patient to ventilator with appropriate mode and alarm settings.
- Suction as required.

Post-procedure

- $EtCO_2$ monitoring
- X-ray to confirm placement of tracheostomy tube
- ABG approximately **after 30 minutes**
- Ensure key-hole dressing is applied.
- Reposition patient's head and neck.
- Check **cuff** pressure (**18–22 mm Hg**)
- Ensure tracheostomy tubes of the **same size** and **one size smaller** with tracheal dilators are at the bedside in the event of an emergency.
- Observe for **early signs** of:
  - Hemorrhage
  - Pneumothorax
  - Pneumomediastinum
  - Wound infection

If a surgical tracheostomy is performed, leave the dressing intact for **24 hours** to prevent potential bleeding and displacement.

A **surgical tracheostomy** is usually indicated when:
- Anatomical landmarks are unidentifiable and/or grossly abnormal.
- Difficult intubation

CHAPTER 15

Protocol for Care of Patient with Tracheostomy Tube

1. Tracheostomy tube with **subglottic suction** should be preferably inserted.
2. Aspirate the subglottic suction port **hourly** to remove any secretions that are collected above the inflated cuff.
3. Emphasis on **hand washing** and **aseptic precautions** prior to tracheostomy care.
4. **Second hourly** suctioning should be done with strict aseptic techniques to clear the airway and ensure tube patency. Any **deviation** in the amount, **color**, and **consistency** of secretions to be notified.
5. Tracheostomy dressing to be done with strict aseptic techniques, **once** in a day and **whenever** necessary.
6. **Oral hygiene** should be maintained with **0.12%** chlorhexidine mouth wash.
7. Secure the tracheostomy tube properly; ensure the **straps** are neither too loose nor too tight.
8. Inspect the **skin** under the securing strap for skin peeling or necrosis.
9. While doing suction, **observe** the patient for hypoxia and vagal stimulation.
10. While feeding a patient with tracheostomy, an **upright position** should be maintained and feeding should be given after back care.

CHAPTER 16

Protocol for Change of Tracheostomy

When a tube is changed, the patient's artificial airway is **temporarily removed**. This should be a planned procedure, carried out by two competent staff. The procedure can be potentially traumatic for the patient, who should be prepared for it.

A skilled practitioner should perform the **first change on day 7**. This is because the stoma and track to the skin from the patient's trachea may not be well formed. In addition, if the tracheostomy has been performed percutaneously the stoma is likely to be tight.

EQUIPMENT

- Ensure all types of emergency equipment are working and ready
- Dressing pack/trolley
- Suitable size tracheostomy (see types of tubes below)
- Sterile water
- **20 mL** syringe
- Sterile gloves
- Keyhole dressing

- Closed suction catheter (appropriate diameter) or single use "Y" catheters
- **"Guidewire" kit** if available
- Lignocaine 2% topical jelly
- End-tidal carbon dioxide ($EtCO_2$) monitor

PROCEDURE

- Inform patients and significant others if applicable
- Ensure enteral feeds are **ceased 6 hours prior** to the procedure and the aspirate nasogastric tube
- Position patient approximately **30°**, head moderately extended
- May enlist physiotherapy treatment prior to the procedure but allow at least **20 minutes** thereafter to prevent potential respiratory embarrassment
- Prepare tracheostomy tube
- **Inflate cuff** and submerge in sterile water to check for leaks, deflate cuff
- Lubricate cuff with Lignocaine **2% jelly** (use of obturator is operator's preference)
- Prepare patient
- **Preoxygenate** with 100% O_2 for 3–5 minutes
- Repeat and inform the patient of the procedure
- Remove old tracheostomy dressing
- Suction lower airway once
- Perform cuff release on second suction
- Deflate the cuff and remove the tracheostomy
- Insertion of new tracheostomy tube

Method 1 (Using Obturator)

- Deflate old tracheostomy and remove the tube
- Rapidly insert a new tube angled at 90° to the trachea, rotate to a downward position (may feel some resistance, especially if it is a percutaneous stoma)
- Inflate the cuff (**18–22 mm Hg**)
- Remove obturator and insert, inner unfenestrated cannula
- Confirm with $EtCO_2$
- Attach to ventilator, check mode and alarm parameters
- Auscultate the chest for air entry and observe chest movement
- Secure tracheostomy and dress appropriately
- Follow-up chest X-ray if applicable

Method 2 (Obturator Not Required)

- A single Y-suction catheter is required for this method or a guidewire kit if available.
- After suctioning leave the **"Y" suction catheter** in situ and cut off the end as this will keep the pathway (a guidewire is used in the same way).
- Deflate cuff and remove old tracheostomy over the catheter or guidewire.
- Guide the new tracheostomy tube over the catheter or guidewire until the correct position is attained, remove catheter or guidewire and inflate the cuff.
- **Follow all other procedures** as for **Method 1**.

Chapter 17: Strategies in ICU to Prevent VAP

1. **Daily oral care** with chlorhexidine mouth wash (0.12% solution) for patients on mechanical ventilator.
2. **Head-end elevation** of alpha beds in ICU: 30–45° to prevent microaspiration of gastric contents.
3. **Intubation with endotracheal** (orotracheal) with subglottic, and also use of tracheostomy tubes with **subglottic suctions** which enable subglottic secretions drainage. Tubes with **ultrathin polyurethane cuff** are desirable.
4. **Stress ulcer prophylaxis** with H_2 receptor blocker or proton pump inhibitor.
5. **Spontaneous awakening** trial with daily sedation interruption, encouraging shorter duration of mechanical ventilation by daily assessment of readiness to wean.
6. Use of **Heat Moisture Exchanger** (passive humidification advocated over active humidifier).
7. **Strict hand hygiene** with chlorhexidine-alcohol solution prior to airway management.
8. Noninvasive ventilation strategy or **high-flow nasal oxygen trial** whenever possible to prevent intubation or reintubation.

9. **Usage of single use/disposable ventilator circuits** (one per patient), routine periodic change not recommended unless visibly soiled.
10. **Closed system suctioning system** not only enables repeated disconnection of a patient from the ventilator, but also prevents aerosolization of organisms.
11. **Insertion of orogastric tube** has provided favorable outcomes as compared to nasogastric tube as ventilator-associated pneumonia (VAP) prevention modality **(level 2 evidence)**.
12. **Appropriate patient-nurse** ratio, meticulous adherence to bundles, hand hygiene practices, nursing education, and periodic audit of implementation of bedside protocols amount to reduction in VAP rate.
13. **Other pharmacological strategies** with level 1 evidence include short course of antibiotics, restriction of blood product usage, influenza, and pneumococcal vaccination.

SECTION 4

Cardiorespiratory Arrest in ICU

18. Adult Tachycardia Algorithm Based on American Heart Association 2020
19. Adult Bradycardia Algorithm Based on American Heart Association 2020
20. Adult Cardiac Arrest Algorithm Based on the Guidelines by American Heart Association 2020
21. Defibrillation Usage in ICU

CHAPTER 18

Adult Tachycardia Algorithm Based on American Heart Association 2020

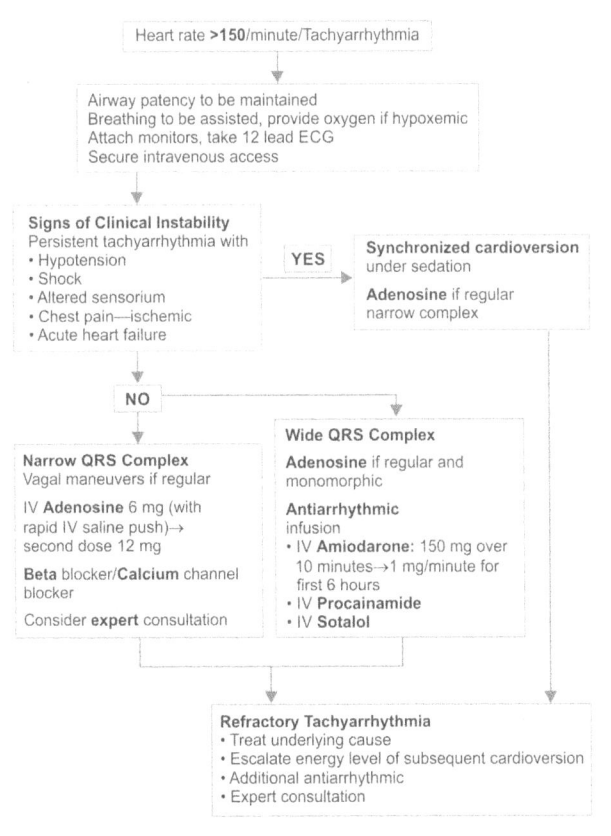

CHAPTER 19

Adult Bradycardia Algorithm Based on American Heart Association 2020

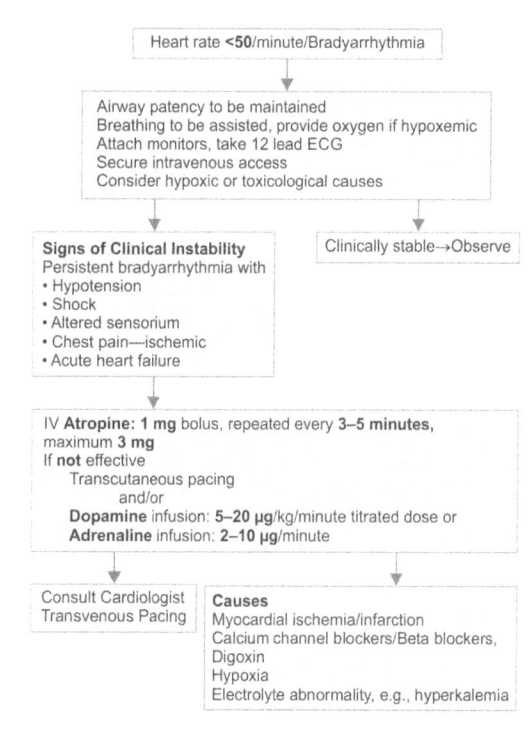

CHAPTER 20

Adult Cardiac Arrest Algorithm Based on the Guidelines by American Heart Association 2020

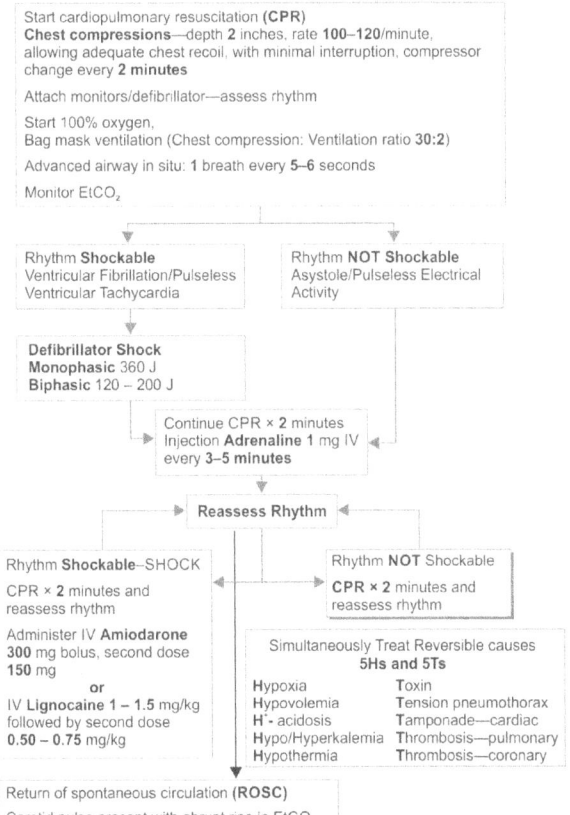

CHAPTER 21: Defibrillation Usage in ICU

PLACEMENT OF PADDLES

1. **Anterior-apex** position maximizes the current flow through the myocardium.
2. Paddles over **infraclavicular** area over right chest.

INDICATIONS

1. To eradicate life-threatening ventricular fibrillation or pulseless ventricular tachycardia.
2. To restore coordinated electric and mechanical pumping action, to improve cardiac output, tissue perfusion, and oxygenation.
3. Synchronized cardioversion in an unstable patient with narrow and wide QRS complex tachyarrhythmias.

EQUIPMENT

1. Defibrillator with electrocardiogram **oscilloscope**
2. Paddles of appropriate diameter (**adult 8.5–12 cm**)
3. Appropriate conductive material gel, conductive paste, remote or hands-free adhesive defibrillation electrodes connected directly to the defibrillator.

4. **Emergency drugs:**
   - Epinephrine—**1 mg** (10 mL—1:10000)
   - 2% Lignocaine (preservative free)—**20 mg**/mL
   - Sodium bicarbonate—**1 mEq**/mL
   - Magnesium—**2 g** (2 mL of 50% solution)
5. Flowmeter for oxygen administration
6. Crash Cart
7. Bag valve mask device (AMBU) or Bain's circuit
8. Emergency suction and intubation equipment
9. Emergency pacing equipment

ASSESSMENT

1. Check carotid pulse.
2. Check monitor for ventricular fibrillation (VF), ventricular tachycardia (VT) pulseless
3. Assess for current ventricular fibrillation
   Biphasic 200 J
   Monophasic 360 J
4. Determine **current arrhythmia** including paroxysmal tachycardia, atrial fibrillation, atrial flutter, atrial tachycardia, and ventricular tachycardia.

PREPARATION

1. Ensure **scene safety**.
2. Ensure **safety** of the patient, away from **metallic objects** and **pooled water**.
3. Assess responsiveness.
4. Call for **help** with defibrillator.
5. Place the patient in **supine** position.

6. **Nitroglycerin (NTG) patch** if preserved should be **removed**.
7. If **Pacemaker** is present, place paddles **2 inches away**.
8. Start **advanced cardiac life support (ACLS) protocol**.

PROCEDURE

1. Switch **on** the defibrillator on the defibrillator mode.
2. Apply the **gel** evenly on the paddles.
3. Position the defibrillator cables to allow adequate **access** to the patient.
4. Turn on **ECG** recorder for continuous print out.
5. Place one paddle at the **apex** of the **heart** on (if **monophasic**).
6. Apply **pressure** to each paddle against the chest wall.
7. State, all clear, **three times** and make sure that all personnel are away from the patient, bed, and equipment.
8. Verify that the patient is still in **ventricular fibrillation** or pulseless **ventricular tachycardia**.
9. Depress both the buttons on the **paddles simultaneously** and **hold defibrillator fire**, there will be an immediate release of electric charges.
10. **Resume cardio-pulmonary resuscitation (CPR) after shock** for **2 minutes** and then assess rhythm and carotid pulse check.

11. Follow the **protocol** of ventricular fibrillations/pulseless ventricular Tachycardiac/Asystole/PEA
12. If successful, obtain vital signs and observe the patient.
13. **Clean the paddles** and **dry**, ensure placement and integrity of electrodes.
14. Discard used supplies and wash hands.

PATIENT MONITORING

1. Evaluate airway, breathing, circulation/intubation, and mechanical ventilation if indicated.
2. Administer **antiarrhythmic** therapy as prescribed. Continue the same antiarrhythmic used during CPR.
3. Assess skin for burn.
4. Monitor ECG.
5. Documentation

SECTION 5

Acid–Base Imbalance and Dyselectrolytemia

22. Sampling of Arterial Blood Gas
23. Steps of Arterial Blood Gases Interpretation
24. Protocol for Potassium Correction in Hypokalemia
25. Protocol for Treatment of Hyperkalemia
26. Hyponatremia Algorithm
27. Protocol for Sodium Correction in Hyponatremia
28. Protocol to Calculate Rate of Infusion for 3% NaCl
29. Protocol for Hypernatremia

CHAPTER 22

Sampling of Arterial Blood Gas

ARTERIAL PUNCTURE—RADIAL ARTERY (PREFERRED)

- Procedure to be explained to conscious cooperative patient.
- Palpate right and left radial artery and select the side with more prominent pulsations suitable for puncture.
- Perform **Allen's test** to determine intactness of collateral circulation by the ulnar artery.

EQUIPMENT [USUALLY PROVIDED IN AN ARTERIAL BLOOD GAS (ABG) SAMPLING KIT]

- A **3–5 mL** preheparinized syringe
  If syringe is not preheparinized, draw **1 mL** of heparin solution (**1:1000** or **1000** IU/mL) into the syringe, moving the plunger up and down a few times to coat the barrel of the syringe. Then **expel** all of the visible heparin through the needle immediately before drawing blood, leaving only a trace of heparin in the needle and in the syringe.
- 25 gauge needle

- Alcohol swabs
- Gauze pad
- Protective equipment for universal precautions

PROCEDURE

1. Procedure done under strict asepsis, use sterile gloves.
2. **Position of hand:** Rest the forearm on comfortable surface in supinated position with **dorsiflexion** of wrist.
3. Radial pulse to be palpated **proximal** to flexor crease (about **2 cm**).
4. Prepare the area with an antiseptic swab and/or an alcohol swab.
5. With your **nondominant** hand, use the **index** and **middle** fingers to locate and trap the radial artery, maintaining control of it in a **1 cm** space between the fingers along the artery.
6. Holding the syringe like at an **angle** of **35–40°** with the needle **bevel up**, enter the skin with the needle **angled** toward the flow of blood, in the space between the fingers controlling the artery.
7. Upon entering the lumen of the artery, blood should flow into the syringe, allowing the syringe to **passively** fill.
8. If **no** blood flows into the syringe, **withdraw slightly** because the needle may have passed through both walls of the vessel. It may be possible to see

the blood **pulsate** into the syringe as it fills; further evidence that the sample is arterial in origin.
9. If **no blood** flows into the syringe, it may be necessary to **slowly withdraw** partially and **redirect** the syringe, using the **palpable pulsation** under the fingers as a guide.
10. After **2–3 mL** of blood has been obtained, withdraw the needle quickly and apply the gauze pad using **firm pressure** at the site for at least **5 minutes**. If the patient has a coagulopathy, **10–15 minutes** of firm pressure is required. The goal is to **avoid** a large hematoma or a possible compartment syndrome.
11. **Remove** any **air bubbles** from the sample by first removing and disposing of the needle, then hold the syringe **upright** and **tapping** the syringe to cause any bubbles to rise. Gently push the plunger to **expel** all the air bubbles. **Cap** the syringe so that it is airtight, and roll it between the hands to mix the contents. Place the **capped syringe** on **ice**.
12. Note the patient name, hospital number, date and time, FiO_2, and body temperature and instantly dispatch to the lab.

COMPLICATIONS

Thrombosis, hematoma, arterial embolism, arterial spasm, arterial insufficiency with tissue loss, infection, hemorrhage, pseudoaneurysm formation, and compartment syndrome.

DRAWING SAMPLE FROM ARTERIAL LINE IN SITU

- Strict asepsis
- Aspirate and discard the heparinized saline present in the extension tubing
- Now aspirate blood **three times** the **capacity** of the **extension** tubing, which is later **reinjected** back to the patient through **venous** line.
- Using a **2-mL** heparinized syringe aspirate slowly **1 mL** of sample for ABG.
- Remove all **air bubbles** from the sample.
- Air bubbles in the sample will cause the O_2 levels to be **elevated** and CO_2 levels to be **lowered**.
- **Flush** the line properly and ensure good trace and clear extension.
- If the sample is **not** analyzed immediately, keep it **air tight** and preserve in **ice pack**.
- **Excess heparin** in the sampling syringe may produce **acidification** of the sample.

CHAPTER 23

Steps of Arterial Blood Gases Interpretation

Step 0: Checking validity of Arterial Blood Gases (ABG)

$$\frac{[H^+] \times [HCO_3]}{[PaCO_2]} = 24$$

$$[H^+] = \frac{24 \times [PaCO_2]}{HCO_3}$$

pH	[H$^+$]
7.00	100
7.10	79
7.20	63
7.30	50
7.40	40
7.50	32
7.60	25

Compare the **expected** pH value with that **derived** on ABG report to ascertain validity

HCO_3^- : Bicarbonate

$PaCO_2$: Partial pressure of **Arterial** Carbon Dioxide

Step 1: Oxygenation status

Calculate the **expected PaO$_2$** (it is generally **5** times the **FiO$_2$**)

Alveolar-arterial (A-a) oxygen gradient = PAO$_2$ – PaO$_2$

$$PAO_2 = PiO_2 - \frac{PaCO_2}{RQ}$$

$$PiO_2 = FiO_2 [P_B - P_{H_2O}]$$

Normal value of **A - a** gradient **10–15** mm Hg

PAO$_2$	Partial pressure of **Alveolar** Oxygen
PiO$_2$	Partial pressure of **Inspired** Oxygen
FiO$_2$	**Fraction** of **Inspired** Oxygen
RQ	Respiratory **Quotient**
P$_B$	**Barometric** Pressure
P$_{H_2O}$	Partial Pressure of **Water**

Step 2: Ventilatory status

Normal **PaCO$_2$**—35 - 45 mm Hg

Step 3: Acid–base status

Identify the **primary** disorder by looking at the **pH**
Normal pH—7.35 - 7.45
pH **7.4** to be considered for **calculation** purpose
pH > 7.40 = Alkalemia
pH < 7.40 = Acidemia

Step 4: Respiratory disorders

If pH and PaCO$_2$ are in **opposite** directions, disorder is **Respiratory**

If the **primary** disorder is **Respiratory** determine if it is a **acute** disorder or a **chronic** disorder, (consider history)

A. In acute respiratory disorder (acidosis or alkalosis)
Change in pH = $0.008 \times (PaCO_2 - 40)$
Expected pH = $7.4 \pm$ change in pH

B. In chronic respiratory disorder (acidosis or alkalosis)
Change in pH = $0.003 \times (PaCO_2 - 40)$
Expected pH = $7.4 \pm$ change in pH

Compare the pH on ABG
If pH on ABG is close to answer "**A**", then it is an **acute** disorder
If pH on ABG is close to answer "**B**", then it is an **chronic** disorder

Calculate Compensation
Standard normal value of HCO_3^- = **24** mEq/L
Standard normal value of $PaCO_2$ = **40** mm Hg

Δ : Difference between Standard and Measured value

Respiratory Acidosis
Acute : $\Delta [HCO_3^-] = \mathbf{0.1}$ mEq/L $\times \Delta PaCO_2$
Chronic : $\Delta [HCO_3^-] = \mathbf{0.35}$ mEq/L $\times \Delta PaCO_2$

Respiratory Alkalosis
Acute : $\Delta [HCO_3^-] = \mathbf{0.2}$ mEq/L $\times \Delta PaCO_2$
Chronic : $\Delta [HCO_3^-] = \mathbf{0.5}$ mEq/L $\times \Delta PaCO_2$

Step 5: Metabolic disorders

I. Metabolic acidosis:

Expected PaCO$_2$ = $[1.5 \times HCO_3] + 8 \pm 2$

Anion Gap = Sodium – (Chloride + Bicarbonate)
Anion gap (AG) = $Na^+ - [Cl^- + HCO_3^-]$
Normal AG = 8 ± 4 mEq/L

Corrected anion gap (AGc)
AGc = AG + [2.5 (4 – Serum Albumin)]

Urinary Anion Gap (UAG) = $(uNa^+ + uK^+) - uCl^-$

Urinary Na$^+$	uNa$^+$
Urinary K$^+$	uK$^+$
Urinary Cl$^-$	uCl$^-$

UAG has been used to roughly estimate whether urine **ammonium** is increased or decreased in the evaluation of **hyperchloremic metabolic** acidosis. It is used to determine etiology of normal anion gap metabolic acidosis with hypokalemia

Negative UAG is seen when there is **increase** in **renal H$^+$ Secretion** e.g. diarrhea

Positive UAG is seen when there is **impaired renal H$^+$ excretion** e.g. distal Renal Tubular Acidosis

II. Metabolic alkalosis:

Expected PaCO$_2$ = $[0.7 \times HCO_3^-] + 21 \pm 2$
Urinary Cl$^-$
- < 20 : Chloride responsive (Extra Cellular Volume depletion)
- > 20 : Chloride resistant (Mineralocorticoid depletion, secondary hyperaldosteronism)

Step 6: Mixed disorders
Gap – Gap ratio

"Gap – Gap" ratio, as term literally suggests, **difference** between the **two gaps** or **differences** between their **measured** values and their **normal** values, which are **"Anion gap"** and **"Bicarbonate"**.

The gap - gap ratio is often used in **diabetic ketoacidosis** [which usually leads to **High anion gap** metabolic acidosis (**HAGMA**)] to determine whether an ongoing metabolic acidosis is due to **ongoing ketoacidosis**, or is due to **isotonic saline infusion** in the resuscitatory period.

In these patients, it is difficult to determine whether the HAGMA is the only process or whether there is **additional process** present such as a **normal anion gap** metabolic process, or a metabolic **alkalosis**.

The first Gap is **Anion Gap**. Its **single normal value** is considered to be **12** for calculation purpose. Hence

$$\Delta \text{AG} = \text{Calculated Anion Gap} - 12$$

The second Gap is **difference** between the value of HCO_3^- obtained from **ABG** and its single normal value i.e. **24**.

$$\Delta HCO_3^- = 24 - \text{measured } HCO_3^-$$

Thus

$$\text{Gap – Gap ratio} = \Delta \text{AG}/\Delta [HCO_3^-]$$
$$= \frac{\text{Anion Gap} - 12}{24 - HCO_3}$$

Gap-Gap ratio	Interpretation
<1	**High** Anion Gap Metabolic Acidosis (**HAGMA**) associated with **Normal** Anion Gap Metabolic Acidosis (**NAGMA**)
1	Isolated or **Pure** High Anion Gap Metabolic **Acidosis** (HAGMA)
>1	High Anion Gap Metabolic Acidosis (HAGMA) associated with metabolic **alkalosis**

HCO_3^- therapy (mmols of bicarbonate):

$$(\Delta HCO_3^-) \times \text{body weight} \times 0.5$$

Or

Base deficit × body weight × **0.33**

Half the calculated dose is given which increases pH by **0.2**

Alkali therapy is indicated if arterial blood pH **drops <7.15 to 7.20**

(**exception:** HCO_3^- concentration **<10 to 12** mEq/L with blood pH **>7.15**)

Chapter 24: Protocol for Potassium Correction in Hypokalemia

Normal limit to be maintained: **4.0–5.0 mEq/L**

Correction required if K^+ = (less than) **<4.0** mEq/L

Daily requirement: 40–120 mEq/day

PREREQUISITES FOR INTRAVENOUS POTASSIUM (K^+) CORRECTION

- Patient should have normal renal function.
- Good urine output (**UOP** >1 mL/kg)
  UOP – Urine output
- Even in the presence of abnormal renal function test with good urine output
- Presence of central venous catheter

If the patient does not have urinary catheter and has **normal** renal function, correct K^+ through the **oral** route.

Correction procedure – K^+ = **3.0–4.0 mEq**

20 mEq KCL (10 mL) + 40 mL normal saline = 50 mL

25 mL/hour = **10 mEq/hour**

If there is **No** urinary catheter: **15 mL (20 mEq/L)** oral syrup/or via nasogastric tube

Patient does **Not** require K^+ correction if K^+ **4–5 mEq/L**

Maintain K$^+$ **above 4 mEq/L** for critically ill patients **unless** contraindicated.

[Normal value – Patient value] × Body Weight × **0.4**]

1 amp KCL = 10 mL = 15% W/v = **1.5 g** = **20 mEq**

Syrup **15 mL** = **20** mEq

Maximum recommended dose is **≤1 mEq/kg/hour** for a few hours in **severe** life-threatening hypokalemia

ECG should be monitored if K$^+$ infusion is >**0.5** mEq/kg/hour

Monitor **urine output**

Potassium preferably to be administered through **Central Venous line (5–20 mEq/hour)**

Hypokalemia increases **Digoxin toxicity**

While giving potassium through **peripheral** line, K$^+$ concentration should **not** be >**20** mEq/L

Concomitant correction of hypomagnesemia should be done

Spot urinary K$^+$ <**15** mEq/L – **nonurinary** cause of hypokalemia

24 hours urinary K$^+$ >**30** mEq/day - **urinary loss** of K$^+$

Chapter 25: Protocol for Treatment of Hyperkalemia

Agent	Dose	Onset of action	K⁺ decline	Mechanism of action	Caution
Ca gluconate	**15–20** mg/kg IV	Immediately	Nil	Cardiac myocyte membrane stabilization	Give via **CVC** preferably, over 10 minutes
Glucose insulin	**50%** Dextrose **2** mL/kg + Regular insulin **0.14** unit/kg	15 minutes	**1** mEq/L	Intracellular shift of K⁺	Blood sugar monitoring
NaHCO$_3$	**1–2** mEq/kg IV	4 hours	**0.5–0.75** mEq/L	Intracellular shift of K⁺	ABG showing metabolic acidosis. Watch for volume overload
Salbutamol	**5–10** mg (nebulized) over 15 minutes	15–30 minutes	**1–1.5** mEq/L	Intracellular shift of K⁺	Watch for tachycardia, blood pressure, blood sugar
Lasix	**1–2** mg/kg IV	30–60 minutes	Variable	Elimination of K⁺ through urine	Monitor blood pressure, intravascular volume status

Contd...

Contd...

Agent	Dose	Onset of action	K⁺ decline	Mechanism of action	Caution
Kayexalate (Sodium polystyrene) is a cation exchange Resin used to treat high levels of potassium in the blood, also called hyperkalemia	**0.25–0.5 g/kg PO/PR**	1–2 hours	**0.5–1 mEq/L**	Decreased K^+ absorption from gut. Kayexalate works by helping body to get rid of extra potassium	May cause hypernatremia, Volume overload, Intestinal necrosis in postoperative patients
Renal replacement therapy		Immediate	Variable	Increased elimination	Postdialysis hyperkalemia may recur

Treat underlying cause, stop K^+ containing fluids.

CHAPTER 26

Hyponatremia Algorithm

HYPONATREMIA

A condition that occurs when the level of sodium in the blood is **too low**. With this condition, the body holds onto **too much water**. This **dilutes** the amount of sodium in blood and causes levels to be **low**.

Features of Hyponatremia

Signs and symptoms of hyponatremia depend on the **value** of serum Sodium and the **rate** of decrease in serum Sodium. Depending on rate of decrease, hyponatremia is classified as **acute** (decrease in sodium over **less** than **48** hours), where **cerebral edema** is likely to be of severe degree. **Gradual** fall in sodium value over **more** than **48** hours is termed as **chronic** hyponatremia.

Signs and Symptoms Based on Rate of Decrease in Sodium

Signs and symptoms	Acute	Chronic
Fatigue, headache, nausea, vomiting	125–130 mEq/L	120–125 mEq/L
Confusion, seizure, coma	120–125 mEq/L	110–120 mEq/L

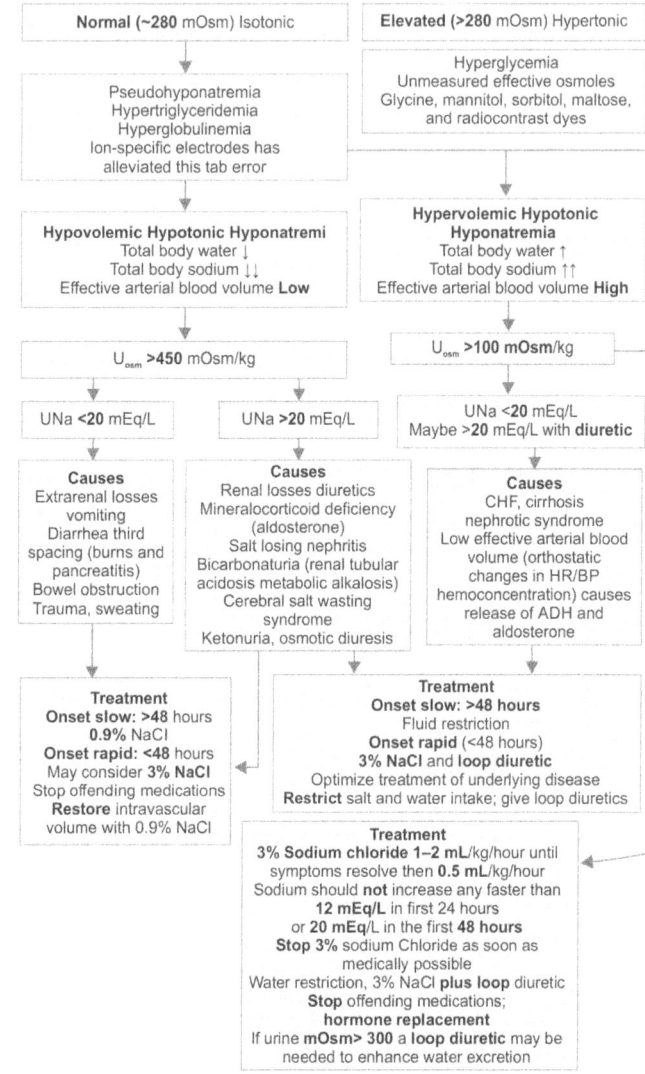

Chapter 26: Hyponatremia Algorithm

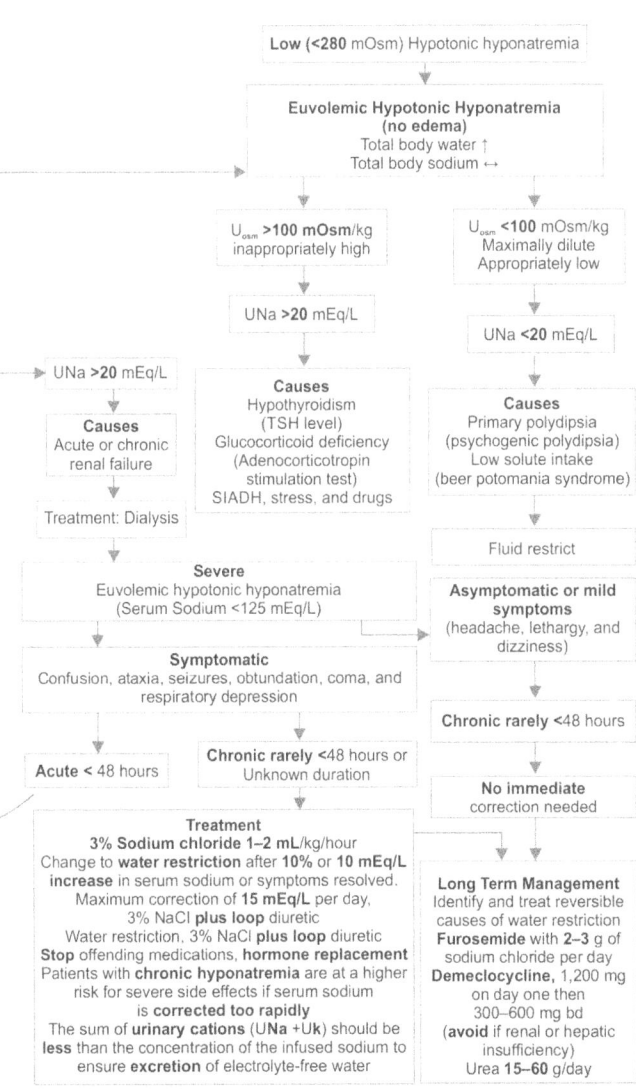

CHAPTER 27

Protocol for Sodium Correction in Hyponatremia

To know **how much** will be the **increase** in serum Na if **1 L** of a particular IV fluid is given.

To find value of **X** refer to following table.

Child	Male	Female	Elderly male	Elderly female
0.6	0.6	0.5	0.5	0.45

TBW = **X** × Body weight (kg)

$$\frac{\text{Concentration of Na in the \textbf{IV fluid} – \textbf{Serum} Na}}{\textbf{TBW} + 1}$$

0.9% NS contains **154** mEq/L of Na

0.9% NS (1 L) given to **60** kg female with Na **110** mEq/L

TBW = 60 × 0.5 = **30** mEq/L

$$\frac{154 - 110}{30 + 1} = \textbf{1.4 mEq/L}$$

1 L of NS will **increase** Na by **1.4** mEq/L.

CHAPTER 28

Protocol to Calculate Rate of Infusion for 3% NaCl

To find value of **X** refer to following table:

Child	Male	Female	Elderly male	Elderly female
0.6	0.6	0.5	0.5	0.45

TBW = X × Body weight (kg)

Na deficit = TBW × [Target Na – Initial Na]

3% NaCl has a **500** mEq/L of Na/L roughly

1 mEq/2 mL

60 kg 60 years female with Na **115 mEq/L**

Goal to increase Na by **8** mEq/L in **24** hours

TBW = 60 × 0.5 = **30** mEq/L

Na deficit = 30 × 123 – 115 = **240**

1 mEq in 2 mL hence **240** mEq in **480** mL

480 mL to be given over **24** hours 480/24 = **20** mL/hour

Hyponatremia which develops rapidly (**acutely**), and is **severe** (**less** than **120** mEq/L) and is symptomatic needs to be corrected rapidly with **3% NaCl**, in order to bring sodium to a safe value (about 125 mEq/L) and to abolish CNS symptoms, after which **slow correction** should be started.

Rapid correction involves administering IV 3% NaCl at **1 mL/kg/h** for **1st 4** hours (**2-3 mL/kg/h** in first 3-4 hours if **active seizure** or signs of **brain herniation**), followed by **slow** correction. Rate of increase in serum Sodium should be **less** than **10-12** mEq/L in first **24** hours or less than **18** mEq/L in initial **48** hours.

If **aggressive** and **rapid** correction is given when it is **not** indicated, it leads to rapid decrease in cerebral edema, resulting in brain shrinkage and demyelination of pontine and extra-pontine neurons. This condition is called as **Osmotic Demyelination Syndrome**, characterized by quadriplegia, pseudo-bulbar palsy, seizure, coma and death.

If there is a **doubt** whether the condition is acute or chronic, then it should be considered to be **chronic** and **slow** correction should be administered.

CHAPTER 29

Protocol for Hypernatremia

CAUSES OF HYPERNATREMIA
- Water deprivation
- Administration of large solute load such as $NaHCO_3$
- Diabetes insipidus
- Excess cortisol production

Measure **electrolytes** and **osmolality** of **plasma** and **urine**

1. **Treat the cause**

2. **Replace** the established water **deficit**

    Water (L) = **0.6 × body weight** in kg $[\{Na_I/Na_F\} - 1]$

    Na_I = **Initial** Na level

    Na_F = **Final** Na level [148 or 20-2.5 mEq/L less than Na_I]

3. **Replace** as **dextrose, 0.45% saline**.

4. Rate of **decrease** of Na should be **1-1.5** mEq/L/h

SECTION 6

General Protocols

30. Protocol for Nutrition in ICU
31. Protocol of Neuromonitoring in ICU
32. Protocol of Glucose Control in ICU
33. Protocol for Bedsore Prevention and Care
34. Protocol for Antibiotic Usage in ICU
35. Protocol for Organ Donor Management

CHAPTER 30: Protocol for Nutrition in ICU

NUTRITIONAL PLAN FOR PATIENT IN INTENSIVE CARE UNIT (ICU)

For example, adult **60 kg** euvolemic, normal urine output, moderate stress

Calculate daily requirement of Energy, Proteins and required fluid volume

Calorie requirement: 25 kcal/kg

$= 25 \times 60$ (wt.) $= 1{,}500$ kcal/day

Protein requirement: 1 g/kg   **1 g Protein** provides 4 kcal

$= 1 \times 60$ (wt.) $= \mathbf{60} \times 4 = 240$ kcal/day

Lipids requirement: 30% of total calorie requirement

$= 30\%$ of $1500 = 450$ kcal/day

1 g lipid provides **9 kcal**

$= 450/9 = \mathbf{50}$ g

Carbohydrates requirement:

= Remaining calorie requirement

$1{,}500 - (240 + 450) = 810$ kcal

1 g carbohydrate provides **4 kcal**

$= 810/4 = \mathbf{202.5}$ g

TOTAL PARENTERAL NUTRITIONAL PRESCRIPTION

$$\text{Fluid volume required} = \frac{\textbf{Amount of substance (g)}}{\textbf{Concentration of substance}} \times 100$$

Proteins: For example, **7% amino acid solution**

$$(\mathbf{60}/7) \times 100 = 857 \text{ mL}$$

Lipids: For example, **10% intralipid solution**

$$(\mathbf{50}/10) \times 100 = 500 \text{ mL}$$

Carbohydrates: For example, **10% dextrose**

$$(\mathbf{202.5}/10) \times 100 = 2{,}025 \text{ mL}$$

ENTERAL NUTRITION

Step 1: Calculate daily requirement of energy and proteins

Step 2: Select feeding formula

Step 3:

$$\text{Feeding volume (mL)} = \frac{\text{kcal/day required}}{\text{kcal/mL in feeding formula}}$$

Step 4: Estimate protein quantity in amount in above calculated feeding volume

Feeding volume (L/day) × Protein (g/L)

In case of **protein intake deficit**, add **supplemental protein**.

GUIDELINES FOR TUBE FEEDING

1. Feeding solutions have to be treated with **hygienic** precautions during preparation, storage, and administration.
2. Feeds should be prepared **fresh** and given **immediately**. Feeds to be **lukewarm**, **Not** too cold, and not too hot.
3. Stream or filter all the feeds before administration in case of blenderized feeds.
4. **Flush** the tube **before** and **after** feeding with clear water.
5. Keep head of bed **elevated 30–45°** during and 30–60° after feed.
6. Record **date** and **time** when the commercial formula is opened. Do **not** use the product after the expiry date.
7. **Avoid** adding colorants, medications, or other substances directly to the formula.
8. If **loose stools** occur, first step is to avoid milk.

CHAPTER 31

Protocol of Neuromonitoring in ICU

PURPOSE

To **prevent secondary brain injury** induced by ischemia, hypoxia, cerebral edema, and metabolic derangements.

1. Patient to be received in intensive care unit (ICU) on alpha beds with side rails. Head to be kept in **neutral, 30° propped up** position with no flexion/rotation.
2. **Glasgow Coma Scale** to be checked **every hour** and any changes in sensorium and pupillary size and reaction immediately reported to neurosurgeon.

	Eye opening		Motor response		Verbal
4	Spontaneously	6	Obeys commands	5	Oriented
3	To verbal stimulus	5	Localizes pain	4	Confused
2	To painful stimulus	4	Withdraws to pain	3	Inappropriate words
1	No eye opening	3	Flexion to pain	2	Incomprehensible sounds
		2	Extension to pain	1	No verbal response
		1	No motor response		

3. Airway protection by endotracheal intubation if indicated (generally if **GCS below 8**), to be done with due consideration to factors that contribute to **rise** in **intracranial pressure (ICP)**.
   - Use of optimal sedation and analgesia
   - Agents to attenuate hemodynamic fluctuation/pressor response to intubation
   - Smooth intubation by experienced operator
   - Avoid succinylcholine raises ICP
   - Preoxygenation to prevent desaturation
   - Simultaneous pharmacological management of ICP
4. Maintain oxygenation, monitor oxygen saturation. Attempt to improve oxygenation by applying **PEEP (positive end-expiratory pressure)** may accelerate ICP.
5. Thorough hemodynamic monitoring, invasive blood pressure monitoring is often preferred.

   Cerebral perfusion pressure (**CPP**)
   Mean arterial pressure (**MAP**)
   Intracranial pressure (**ICP**)

   $$CPP = MAP - ICP$$

   Maintain CPP = **50–70** mm Hg

   Normal ICP <**15** mm Hg

   Raised ICP >**20** mm Hg

   a. **Prevent hypotension** to allow adequate cerebral perfusion, and treat with adequate fluid administration and use of **noradrenaline infusion** to achieve target MAP.

b. **Hypertension** to be treated with intravenous (IV) **labetalol** or **nicardipine**. **Avoid** nitroglycerine which raises ICP.
c. **Judicious use of IV fluids** to be practiced. Euvolemia to be maintained. Use iso-/hyperosmolar nondextrose containing fluids. IV **0.9% normal saline (NS)** is **preferred**, but may cause normal anion gap metabolic acidosis. **Ringer lactate (RL)** has a drawback of being relatively **hypoosmolar**. **NS** and **RL** may be **alternated** to counteract each of the drawbacks.

6. **Sedation** should be administered to reduce/maintain normal ICP, decrease metabolic demands, prevent fluctuations in blood pressure, and avoid coughing and bucking by patient and not allowing patient-ventilator dyssynchrony.

   Agents of choice are propofol, fentanyl, midazolam, dexmedetomidine, and thiopentone.

7. **Maintain normal body temperature**. Core temperature monitoring may be warranted.
   - **Fever to be treated** with surface cooling and administration of IV paracetamol. Fever may trigger secondary brain injury by increasing metabolic demands.
   - In case of **hypothermia**, use warm blankets, body warmer, and administration of warm IV fluids.

8. Watch for **Cushing's triad**
   Hypertension, bradycardia, and respiratory depression, signifying raised ICP.
   - **Use of hyperventilation**
     Acute rise in ICP can be treated by hyperventilating, which leads to a brief decrease in ICP. End-tidal carbon dioxide ($EtCO_2$) to be maintained between **26 and 30 mm Hg**.
   - **IV mannitol 20% administration**
     1 g/kg followed by **0.25–0.5 g/kg 6–8 hourly** decreases ICP by virtue of being osmotic diuretic. Consider patient's renal and cardiac functioning prior to administration. Monitoring of blood pressure, serum electrolytes namely sodium, potassium, magnesium, serum osmolality, and serum creatinine is essential during ongoing therapy.
   - **IV Lasix (furosemide) 0.5–1** mg/kg
     Loop diuretic may be useful in reducing ICP. Monitor Sr K, blood pressure, and intravascular volume status.
   - **3% NaCl**
     Alternatively, IV bolus of **3%** NaCl over **15–20 minutes** attenuates rise in ICP, which can be repeated at 8 hours of interval. Serum Na to be monitored every **8–12** hours and maintained between **140 and 145** mEq/L.
   - **IV dexamethasone**
     IV dexamethasone **helps with raised** ICP secondary to intracranial tumor or infection.

- **Glycerol administration**
  Glycerol administration is believed to **enable faster** but **less effective** reduction in ICP.
9. Definitive causes of **rise in ICP should be treated**. Decompressive craniotomy, evacuation of clot, tumor resection, and insertion of external ventricular drain are surgical options to consider.
10. **Prophylactic anticonvulsant** administration if indicated.
11. **Invasive ICP monitoring** is indicated in the following situations:
    - GCS 3–8 with **abnormal CT** finding
    - GCS 3–8 with **normal CT** finding
      a. If age >40 years, unilateral or bilateral posturing
      b. Systolic blood pressure <90 mm Hg

CHAPTER 32
Protocol of Glucose Control in ICU

Patients in intensive care unit (ICU) admitted with critical illnesses require **cessation** of all **oral hypoglycemic agents** and **subcutaneous insulin** and management of blood sugars is to be done with **intravenous (IV) regular insulin** [half-life $(t_{1/2})$—**5-9 minutes**].

Target blood glucose (BG) level range: 140–180 mg/dL

INSULIN INFUSION

1 unit/mL infusion (diluted with **0.9% NaCl**) administered intravenously via **infusion pump. Prime** the IV tubing by flushing initial infusion through it before connecting to IV line.

BOLUS AND INITIAL INFUSION RATE

Divide initial BG by **70**, **round** it to the nearest 0.5 units

- This amount **"x"** should be given as **IV bolus** (caution in individuals with **creatinine >2**)
- Start infusion at the **same rate** ("x" mL/h)
- **NO** bolus dose is required if initial BG is **<180 mg/dL**

MONITORING

- Blood glucose is to be monitored **1 hourly** with glucometer (**capillary blood**) until **3 consecutive** readings are in target range following which one can monitor BG **2 hourly**.
- Resume **1 hourly monitoring** if insulin rate is changed, if there is **worsening** of hemodynamic/clinical status of patient, change in requirement of vasopressor/inotropes, steroids, or alteration in nutritional support and during dialysis.

Change the insulin infusion rate based on the following suggested algorithm:

1. Identify BG value of previous hour (**BG1**).
2. Check the blood sugar after **1 hour** of resumption of insulin infusion. Consider this value to be **BG2**.
3. On basis of the **value of BG2**, refer to the following table and decide the column number (**namely 1, 2, 3, and 4**).
4. After identifying column number, calculate the **difference** between present BG value (**BG2**) and that of the previous hour (**BG1**) to obtain the change in BG value in 1 hour.
   If checked **after 2** hours, divide this value **by 2**.
5. Based on change in BG, identify the "**Instructions**" in the last column, where Δ = rate of change of insulin infusion (units per hour).

Determine the Rate of Change from Prior Blood Glucose

BG 100–130	BG 140–179	BG 180–249	BG > 250	Instructions
		BG **increased** by **>40** mg/dL	BG **increased**	**Increase Drip by 2 Δ**
	BG **increased** by **>20** mg/dL/h	BG **increased** by **1–40** mg/L/h or BG **unchanged**	BG **unchanged** or BG **decreased** by **1–40** mg/dL/h	**Increase Drip by Δ**
Blood glucose (**BG**) **increased**	BG **increased** by **1–20** mg/dL Or BG **unchanged** Or BG **decreased** by **1–20** g/dL/h	BG **decreased** by **1–40** mg/dL	BG **decreased** by **41–80** mg/dL/h	**NO D**rip change
BG **unchanged** or **decreased** by **1–20** mg/dL/h	BG **decreased** by **21–40** mg/dL/h	BG **decreased** by **41–80** mg/dL/h	BG **decreased** by **80–120** mg/dL/h	**Decrease Drip by Δ**
BG **decreased** by **>20** mg/dL/h	BG **decreased** by **>40** mg/dL/h	BG **decreased** by **>80** mg/dL/h	BG **decreased** by **>120** mg/dL/h	Hold **D**rip for **30 minutes** and then **decrease D**rip by **2 Δ**

6. To obtain the **value of "Δ"**, refer to the following table:

Current rate of infusion (Unit/h)	Δ = rate of change (Units/h)	2 Δ (Units/h)
<3	0.5	1
3–6	1	2
6.5–9.5	1.5	3
10–14.5	2	4
15–19.5	3	6
20–24.5	4	8
>25	5	10

7. **Derive the** new rate of infusion and **repeat** the above steps for the subsequent hours.

MANAGEMENT OF HYPOGLYCEMIA

1. If BG is between **60 and 80** mg/dL—**stop insulin** infusion and give IV **25% dextrose 50 mL** (100 mL if BG is <60 mg/dL).
2. Recheck BG in **15 minutes** until BG is >110 mg/dL.
3. Assess need for restarting insulin infusion in consultation with physician.

SWITCHING OVER TO SUBCUTANEOUS INSULIN REGIMEN

1. Switch to **subcutaneous insulin** once **euglycemic** and hemodynamically stable for at least **24 hours** with consistent dietary intake and suitable for discharge from ICU.

2. Give **short-acting insulin subcutaneously** at **two times** the drip rate along with **0.3 U/kg** of **long acting insulin** and then **turn off** the infusion drip immediately.
3. If **short-acting** insulin is **NOT** administered, then overlap **long-acting insulin** with the insulin **infusion** for **2–4 hours** in order to prevent **rebound hyperglycemia**.

CHAPTER 33: Protocol for Bedsore Prevention and Care

1. Identify patient **at risk** of developing pressure sore/bedsore:
   - Comorbid conditions which impair microcirculation:
     - Diabetes mellitus
     - Peripheral vascular disease
     - Cerebrovascular accident
     - Malignancy, decreased body mass index (BMI)
   - Sepsis, septic shock
   - Age >70 years
   - Chronic smoking
   - Pre-existing poor nutritional status, poor hydration
   - Immobility
   - Fecal and urinary incontinence

2. At admission in critical care unit, examine patient for **presence** of pressure sore or skin changes and document:
   - Location
   - Size
   - Number of days with pressure ulcer if known
   - Category/stage (**refer table**)

Category/stage	Description
I	Nonblanchable erythema
II	Partial thickness skin loss—epidermis, dermis involved
III	Full thickness skin loss—involves subcutaneous tissue
IV	Full thickness tissue loss—muscle and bone
	Unstageable: Depth unknown

3. **Preventive measures** to be implemented at admission. Nursing education regarding preventive measures of bedsores is of paramount importance.

4. **Daily assessment** of skin should be done for early identification of skin breakdown and early enforcement of curative measures.

5. **Frequent turning** and **position change** should be done at **4 hourly interval**, except at night. These positions include supine, left partial lateral, and right partial lateral.

Pressure Points in each Position Prone for Development of Pressure Sore

Supine	Lateral	Prone
Occiput	Ear, cheek, and side of the head	Elbow, ear, cheek, and nose
Scapula	Acromion process	Breasts (female)
Elbow	Elbow	Genitalia (male)
Sacrum/buttock	Trochanter	Iliac crest
Heels	Medial and lateral condyle	Patella
	Medial and lateral malleolus	Toes

6. Use **viscoelastic** foam mattresses or **air** mattresses which enable redistribution of pressure over greater surface rather than a single pressure point, thus preventing sores.

7. **Nutritional support** and **rehabilitation** play a vital role in both prevention and management of pressure sore. **Albumin** level **<3.5** is postulated to be a risk factor for ulcer development and for nonhealing ulcer. Protein supplementation (**1.25–1.5 g/kg/day**), minerals and trace elements supplementation may benefit in **case deficiency** is suspected.

8. Over a pressure sore, cleaning should be done with nontoxic solution, **normal saline** 0.9% being **preferred** solution. **Povidone iodine** has been found to be toxic to fibroblasts.

9. **Debridement** of necrotic tissue promotes wound healing. Opinion of surgeon should be sought for better management.

10. Look for **signs of secondary wound infection** such as pus/exudates, foul odor, delayed wound healing. Pus swab should be taken and meticulous dressing should be done. Silver sulfadiazine or silver impregnated dressings are found to be effective in decreasing bacterial load. Topical/oral antibiotics may be used.

11. Dressing should be done with **nonadherent** dressing or a foam dressing.

12. **Analgesic** should be administered **prior** to dressing change in case of severe pain.

13. **Adjuvant therapeutic modalities** such as hyperbaric oxygen, negative pressure wound therapy, and electrical stimulation may be implemented.

14. **Monitoring of healing of ulcer** has to be done and documented.

CHAPTER 34: Protocol for Antibiotic Usage in ICU

S. No.	Condition	Risk factor	Antibiotic		Duration
1.	Community-acquired pneumonia in ICU	No risk factor for *Pseudomonas aeruginosa* infection	**Non-pseudomonal beta-lactam**	Cefotaxime	7–10 days
				Ceftriaxone	
			plus		
			Macrolide	Azithromycin	
				Clarithromycin	
			or		
			Respiratory fluoroquinolone	Levofloxacin	**Allergic to Penicillin**
				Moxifloxacin	
				Ciprofloxacin	
			and		
			Aztreonam		

Contd...

Chapter 34: Protocol for Antibiotic Usage in ICU

Contd...

S. No.	Condition	Risk factor	Antibiotic		Duration
1.	Community-acquired pneumonia in ICU	**Risk factor** for *Pseudomonas aeruginosa* Chronic pulmonary disease Systemic steroids Elderly Immunocompromised Prior use of antibiotic Enteral feeding tube CVA Cardiovascular disease	**Antipneumococcal and antipseudomonal antibiotic**		14 days
			Beta-lactam	Ceftazidime	
				Cefoperazone	
				Piperacillin	
				Tazobactam	
				Cefoperazone	
				Sulbactam	
				Cefepime	
			Carbapenem	Imipenem	
				Meropenem	
			may add		
			Aminoglycoside	Amikacin	
			or		
			Antipseudomonal fluoroquinolone	Ciprofloxacin	
		Risk for MRSA (methicillin-resistant *Staphylococcus aureus*)		Vancomycin	14–21 days
				Teicoplanin	

Contd...

Contd...

S. No.	Condition	Risk factor	Antibiotic		Duration
1.	**Community-acquired pneumonia in ICU**	**VRSA** Vancomycin-resistant *Staphylococcus Aureus*, or renal failure		Linezolid	14–21 days
		Anaerobic coverage Aspiration Altered sensorium		Piperacillin Tazobactam Carbapenem cover anaerobe	
		Lung abscess Empyema Necrotizing pneumonia	**may add**	Amoxicillin-clavulanate Clindamycin Moxifloxacin	

Contd...

Contd...

S. No.	Condition	Risk factor	Antibiotic		Duration
2.	Ventilator-associated pneumonia	**Not at risk of** Multidrug-resistant organisms **(MDR)** or **MRSA/ Hospitalized for <5 days**	**Third-generation cephalosporin**	Ceftriaxone	7–8 days
			or		
			Ampicillin Sulbactam		
			or		
			Respiratory Fluoroquinolone	Levofloxacin	
				Moxifloxacin	
			or		
			Non-antipseudomonal carbapenem	Ertapenem	
		MDR organisms, *Pseudomonas*	**Antipseudomonal Cephalosporin**	Cefepime	14 days
				Ceftazidime	
			or		
			Antipseudomonal Carbapenem	Imipenem	
				Meropenem	
			or		
			Antipseudomonal Penicillin with Beta-lactamase inhibitor	Piperacillin Tazobactam	
				Ceftazidime-Avibactam	

Contd...

Contd...

S. No.	Condition	Risk factor	Antibiotic		Duration
2.	Ventilator-associated pneumonia		**plus**		
		MDR organisms, *Pseudomonas*	**Aminoglycoside**	Amikacin	
				Gentamycin	
				Tobramycin	
			plus		
		MRSA	**Anti-MRSA agent**	Linezolid	
				Teicoplanin	
				Vancomycin	
				Ceftaroline	
		VAP with atypical organism (5–7.5%)	**Macrolide**	Azithromycin	
				Clarithromycin	
			or		
			Respiratory fluoroquinolone	Levofloxacin	
				Moxifloxacin	

S. No.	Condition	Risk factor	Antibiotic	Duration
3.	Central line-associated blood stream infection	**Gram positive**	**Vancomycin, Teicoplanin**	14 days
		Coagulase-negative Staphylococcus (CONS)	**Alternative: Linezolid, Daptomycin**	7 days
		MRSA		14 days
		Complicated infection		4–6 weeks

Contd...

Contd...

S. No.	Condition	Risk factor	Antibiotic		Duration
3.	Central line-associated blood stream infection	Gram-negative coverage	Fourth-generation cephalosporin	Cefepime	7 days
			or		
			Beta-lactam with beta-lactamase inhibitor (BLBLI)	Piperacillin–tazobactam	
			or		
			Carbapenem	Meropenem	
			±		
			Aminoglycoside	Amikacin	
		Candida	Echinocandin	Anidulafungin	14 days
			or		
			Azole	Fluconazole	
4.	Catheter-associated urinary tract infection	ESBL gram negative, (extended-spectrum beta-lactamase)	Aminoglycoside		
			BLBLI		
			Carbapenem		
5.	Acute infective diarrhea	*Clostridium difficile*	Metronidazole		10–14 days
			Vancomycin		

Contd...

Contd...

S. No.	Condition	Risk factor	Antibiotic		Duration
6.	Peritonitis in ICU	Primary peritonitis	**Third-generation cephalosporin**	Cefotaxime Ceftriaxone	7–10 days
		Secondary peritonitis	**BLBLI**		4 days after adequate source control/ surgery
			Carbapenem		
			with anaerobic cover	Metronidazole	
7.	Skin and soft tissue infection in ICU	Nonpurulent		Clindamycin	
		Severe nonpurulent	**BLBLI**	Piperacillin-Tazobactam	
			plus		
			MRSA cover	Vancomycin Teicoplanin Linezolid Daptomycin	
		Severe purulent	**Incision and drainage with BLBLI plus MRSA cover**		5 days
		Necrotizing fasciitis	**BLBLI**		2–3 weeks
			plus		
			Fluoroquinolone		
			plus		
			anaerobic cover	Clindamycin	

Contd...

Contd...

S. No.	Condition	Risk factor	Antibiotic		Duration
8.	**Sepsis of unknown cause in ICU**	Community-acquired	**Third-generation cephalosporin**	Ceftriaxone	7–10 days
			plus		
			Macrolide	Clarithromycin	
			or		
			Doxycycline		
		Hospital-acquired	**BLBLI**		7–10 days
			plus		
			Fluoroquinolone		
			or		
			Aminoglycoside		

9.	**Meningitis in ICU**	**Community-acquired meningitis**			
		Empirical	**Third-generation cephalosporin**		14 days
		Streptococcus pneumoniae	plus		
			Vancomycin		
		>50 years, immunocompromised	**add ampicillin or amoxicillin**		
		Listeria monocytogenes	**Ampicillin** **Sulfamethoxazole/** **Trimethoprim in Penicillin allergy**		≥21 days

Contd...

Contd...

S. No.	Condition	Risk factor	Antibiotic		Duration
9.	**Meningitis in ICU**	*Neisseria meningitidis*	**Ampicillin**		7 days
			Ceftriaxone		
		Herpes encephalitis	**Acyclovir**		14 days
		Nosocomial meningitis			
		Empirical	Cefepime or Ceftazidime		
			or		
			Meropenem		
		Acinetobacter	Colistin		21 days
		Brain abscess			
			Third-generation cephalosporin		4 weeks minimum
			plus		
			Metronida-zole		
		MRSA	**plus**		
			Vancomycin		
		Beta-lactam contra-indicated	**Ciprofloxacin plus Vancomycin**		
		Ciprofloxacin contra-indicated	**Aztreonam**		

Contd...

Contd…

S. No.	Condition	Risk factor	Antibiotic		Duration
10.	**Invasive fungal infection (in non-neutropenic patients)**	Empirical therapy for patients at risk	**Fluconazole**		2 weeks
		Risk factors	**or**		
		Surgery	Echino-candins	Caspo-fungin	
		Total parenteral nutrition			
		Renal replacement therapy		**Alternative**	
		Diabetes mellitus			
		Central venous catheter			
		Urinary catheter			
		Candida colonization index >0.5		Micafungin/ Anidula-fungin	
		Acute kidney injury			
		Broad-spectrum antibiotic			
		Mechanical ventilation > 3 days			
		APACHE II score >16			

35. Protocol for Organ Donor Management

After brain death diagnosis focus is on the **support**, **protection,** and **function improvement** of the organs.

Brain death is characterized by **two hemodynamic phases**:

First: This phase is characterized by:
- Massive sympathetic discharge (**autonomic storm**)
- Acute hypertensive crisis
- Severe cardiovascular disturbances

Second: Results from **reduction in sympathetic tone:**
- Deterioration of inotropic and chronotropic status
- Leads to fall in cardiac output

1. **Hemodynamic status:**

Arterial hypotension
↓
Reduced release of catecholamines
↓
Vasodilatation
↓
Decreased peripheral vascular resistance

Hypovolemia due to previous fluid restriction and polyuria due to antidiuretic hormone (ADH) deficiency and hyperglycemia will lead to **hypotension.**

Deterioration of inotropic and chronotropic status due to hormone deficiency (thyroxin, cortisol, vasopressin, and insulin) and anaerobic metabolism leads to **drop** in cardiac output.

Goals of hemodynamic management:
　Maintain adequate circulating volume
　Normal cardiac output
　Good perfusion pressure

Essential to keep systolic blood pressure **(SBP)**
　SBP > 100 mm Hg:
　SBP 80–90 can lead to acute tubular necrosis
　SBP <80 can lead to post-transplant failure (liver)

2. **Electrolyte and fluid balance**
　They are prone for:
　　Free water and electrolyte losses leads to
　　Hypernatremia
　　Hypocalcemia
　　Hypomagnesemia
　　Hypokalemia
　　Hypophosphatemia

Above **factors** make them **prone** for arrhythmias, myocardial dysfunction, and sudden cardiac arrest

a. **Expand plasma volume:**
　Maintain CVP **10–15** cmH$_2$O

Losses in plasma volume occur due to:
Polyurea (ADH deficiency), osmotic diuresis (hyperglycemia), and hyperthermia to be replaced.

b. **Fluid replacement:**
Use **isotonic crystalloid** at a rate of: **5 mL**/kg/hr
Keep **SBP >100** mm Hg or **CVP >12** cmH$_2$O
Blood components: Target hemoglobin **9–10 g/dL**
Avoid pulmonary edema, cardiac overload, and hepatic congestion
Restore normovolemia before starting vasoactive drugs

c. **Vasoactive drugs**
Dopamine is the drug of choice, but in a dose >10 µ/kg/min consider adding **dobutamine**
Noradrenaline if hypotension persists
Vasopressin and **adrenaline** (0.1 µ/kg/min) in desperate cases

d. There are possible beneficial effects of **esmolol** during autonomic storm, hence it may be used to manage hemodynamics.

e. **Monitoring**
CVP, ECHO, pulmonary arterial catheter, cardiac output monitoring [Pulse index Continuous Cardiac Output (PiCCO)], mixed venous oxygen saturation (SvO$_2$), base excess, and lactate

3. **Arrhythmias and conduction disorders**
   Bradycardia (**Cushing's phenomenon**)
   No response to atropine (**nucleus ambiguous destroyed**)
   Isoprenaline recommended (**1–3 μ/min**)

   Causes
   Electrolyte imbalance
   Hypothermia
   Myocardial infarction
   Iatrogenic
   Central origin

   Management
   Correct underlying cause first
   Amiodarone is the first choice
   Refractory ventricular arrhythmias—suspect hypothermia
   Consider QT lengthening
   Discontinue suspected medication, correct dyselectrolytemia, and temporary pacemaker

4. **Temperature control**
   After brain death, hypothalamic control of temperature is lost, hence there is progressive loss of body heat

   Management
   Heated IV solutions to be administered
   Humidification and heating of respiratory gases

Electric blanket (core body temperature to be kept >35°C)

Always prevent hypothermia rather than treating

5. **Diabetes insipidus**

   Very common:

   Occurs as a result of **ADH deficiency**

   There is **Loss** of hypothalamic pituitary control of secretions

   Hence **uncontrolled** increase of hypoconcentrated urine

   Diuresis >**4 mL**/kg/h

   Urine specific gravity **<1.005**

   Plasma osmolarity >**300 mOsm**/kg

   Urinary osmolarity <**300 mOsm**/kg

   Hypernatremia

   Hypomagnesemia

   Hypokalemia

   Hypocalcemia

   Hypophosphatemia

   Treatment

   a. Fluid and ion supplementation to be given
   b. **ADH analogues** if diuresis >**200–250 mL/h**
      Desmopressin (drug of choice)
      IV bolus: 0.03–0.15 µ/kg/8–12 h (1–5 µ/8–12 h)
      Intranasal: 5–40 µ 6 hourly
      Vasopressin is dose dependent
      V_2 effect **1–2 U/h; 2–10 mU**/kg/min

6. **Pituitary disorders**

    Several theories have been postulated as causative

    T_3 administration **stops** anaerobic metabolism

    Sick euthyroid syndrome

    Hormone cocktail (T_3, vasopressin, and methylprednisolone) is administered to counteract hypothalamopituitary failure.

7. **Glucose abnormalities**

    Causes

    Hypersecretion of adrenal hormones
    Catecholamine administration
    Glucocorticoid administration
    Glucose containing solutions
    Hypothermia
    Changes in pancreatic microcirculation

    Implications

    Metabolic acidosis
    Osmotic diuresis
    Hypovolemia
    Dehydration

    Management:

    Continuous IV Insulin with 1-2 hourly blood glucose monitoring to titrate rate of infusion

8. **Ventilatory support**

   Up to **15%** of donors are affected by ARDS due to:

   a. **Catecholamine storm** leading to capillary permeability changes/capillary leakage and hemodynamic alterations

   b. **Inflammatory mediators:**

   Goals:

   PaO_2 >**100 mm Hg** with lowest FiO_2 and PEEP possible, lower minute volume needed

   In Lung transplant:

   Low FiO_2 to avoid oxygen toxicity

   PEEP between **8 and 10** cmH_2O

   Tidal volume **6–8** mL/kg IBW

   Closed circuit for tracheal suction

   Apnea test in CPAP mode

   Recruitment maneuvers after any disconnection

9. **Coagulopathy**

   Multifactorial etiology:

   Ischemic brain leads to release of fibrinolytic agents

   NSAIDs

   Warfarin

   May need FFP, platelets to correct coagulopathy

10. **Infectious complications**

    RS: VAP, aspiration

    Trauma causing localized infections

    Catheters (CVC, arterial, and urinary)

11. Nutrition

Enteral or parenteral
Glucose solutions may be administered

12. Intraoperative management

Care must be continued till organ retrieval

Rule of 100
SBP >100 mm Hg
Urine output >100 mL/h
PaO_2 >100 mm Hg
Hb >100 g/L (10 g/dL)

Keep operation theatre temperature **adequate**

Reflex movements: **Lazarus sign**
Possible due to surgical stimulus
Use neuromuscular blocking agents

Sweating, tachycardia, and hypertension
Stimulation of adrenal medulla by spinal reflex
Analgesic may prevent hemodynamic instability

Reserve of blood products

SECTION 7: Key Points in Ventilating Common ICU Admissions

36. Key Points in Ventilating Respiratory Failure
37. Key Points in Ventilating Postoperative (Normal Lung) Patient
38. Key Points in Ventilating Neuromuscular Diseases
39. Key Points in Ventilating Head/Brain Injury
40. Key Points in Ventilating Severe Asthma
41. Key Points in Ventilating Chronic Obstructive Pulmonary Disease
42. Key Points in Ventilating Acute Respiratory Distress Syndrome
43. Key Points in Care of Patients on Long-term Mechanical Ventilator
44. Ventilator Troubleshooting
45. Weaning Criteria

CHAPTER 36: Key Points in Ventilating Respiratory Failure

TYPES OF RESPIRATORY FAILURE

Type 1	Type 2	Type 3	Type 4
Hypoxemic respiratory failure	Hypercapnic respiratory failure	Perioperative respiratory failure	Shock with hypoperfusion
PaO_2 is **low** <**50** mm Hg	PaO_2 is **low** <**50** mm Hg	FRC falls **below** (**CV**) closing volume leading to atelectasis due to **contributory** factors presents in a patient in **perioperative** period namely • Supine position • Due to general anesthesia • Impaired cough reflex • Pain leading to splinting	**Hypoperfusion** of respiratory muscles in shock
$PaCO_2$ is **Not** elevated	$PaCO_2$ is **elevated** >**60** mm Hg		

Contd...

Contd...

Type 1		Type 2		Type 3	Type 4
Signs and symptoms		**Signs and symptoms**			
1	**Signs of respiratory compensation:** Tachypnea, accessory muscle use Nasal flaring, intercostals Suprasternal, and supraclavicular indrawing	1	**CNS depression:** Drowsiness, confusion, headache flapping tremors, and seizures		
2	**Signs of increased sympathetic tone** tachycardia, hypertension, and sweating	2	Tachycardia, bounding pulse		
		3	Stimulation of respiratory center		
3	**End-organ hypoxia** altered sensorium, cold clammy peripheries	4	**CVS depression** peripheral vasodilatation **(except** pulmonary) flushing, sweating, and warm extremities		
4	Cyanosis				

GOALS OF MECHANICAL VENTILATION

1. **Correct oxygenation**
   SpO_2 >**90%** with **minimum** fraction of inspired oxygen (FiO_2), positive end-expiratory pressure (PEEP) titration, increasing functional residual capacity, and recruitment to enable efficacious gaseous exchange

2. **Permissive hypercapnia**
   $PaCO_2$ >**50** with **pH >7.2**) by use of pressure limited ventilation with low-tidal volume strategy (**6-8** mL/kg) and **Not** allowing P_{plat} (plateau pressure) >**30** cmH_2O and P_{peak} (peak inspiratory pressure) >**35** cmH_2O

3. Implement **early** spontaneous breathing trials. **Avoid prolonged** sedation and paralysis.

Section 7: Key Points in Ventilating Common ICU Admissions

APPROACH TO RESPIRATORY FAILURE
OXYGEN THERAPY/TRIAL OF NIV/HFNO

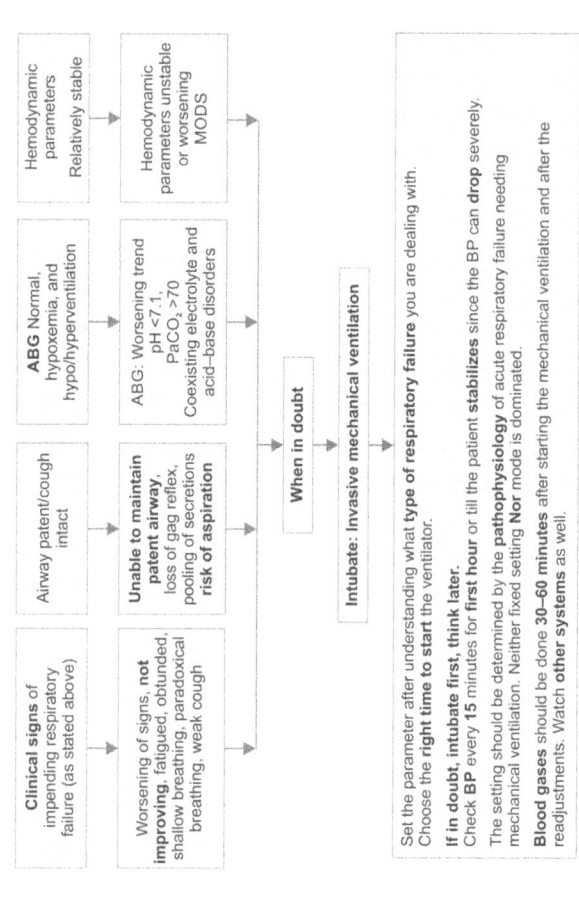

- Clinical signs of impending respiratory failure (as stated above)
- Airway patent/cough intact
- ABG Normal, hypoxemia, and hypo/hyperventilation
- Hemodynamic parameters Relatively stable

- Worsening of signs, **not improving**, fatigued, obtunded, shallow breathing, paradoxical breathing, weak cough
- **Unable to maintain patent airway**, loss of gag reflex, pooling of secretions **risk of aspiration**
- ABG: Worsening trend pH <7.1, PaCO$_2$ >70 Coexisting electrolyte and acid–base disorders
- Hemodynamic parameters unstable or worsening MODS

When in doubt

Intubate: Invasive mechanical ventilation

- Set the parameter after understanding what **type of respiratory failure** you are dealing with. Choose the **right time to start** the ventilator.
- **If in doubt, intubate first, think later.**
- Check **BP** every 15 minutes for **first hour** or till the patient **stabilizes** since the BP can **drop** severely.
- The setting should be determined by the **pathophysiology** of acute respiratory failure needing mechanical ventilation. Neither fixed setting **Nor** mode is dominated.
- **Blood gases** should be done **30–60 minutes** after starting the mechanical ventilation and after the readjustments. Watch **other systems** as well.

Chapter 36: Key Points in Ventilating Respiratory Failure

SUMMARY OF MANAGEMENT OF RESPIRATORY FAILURE

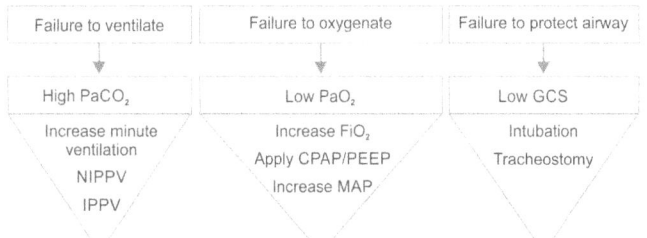

Failure to ventilate	Failure to oxygenate	Failure to protect airway
High $PaCO_2$	Low PaO_2	Low GCS
Increase minute ventilation	Increase FiO_2	Intubation
NIPPV	Apply CPAP/PEEP	Tracheostomy
IPPV	Increase MAP	

Key Points in Ventilating Postoperative (Normal Lung) Patient

CHAPTER 37

Following surgical procedures performed under general anesthesia, reversal from anesthesia is often deferred electively and decision to delay extubation is taken on case to case basis by anesthesiologist due to either the nature of surgery, patient's pre/intraoperative condition, or due to an anticipated postoperative complication.

INDICATIONS FOR ELECTIVE VENTILATION
- Hemodynamic instability
- Brainstem handling
- Preoperative lower cranial palsy
- Massive blood loss
- Intraoperative acute brain bulge
- Residual tumor
- Prolonged surgery **(>8 hours)**
- Not obeying commands
- Airway compromise due to edema or bleeding
- Inadequate pulmonary reserve postsurgery
- Compromised myocardial function expected large fluid shifts with thoracoabdominal procedures
- Continued bleeding with likelihood of return to operating room

These individuals often have a **normally functioning lung**, hence **normal lung physiology** should be **preserved** while delivering invasive positive pressure ventilation.

GOALS OF VENTILATION

1. Enable controlled or assist controlled ventilation for a period of time until patient is deemed suitable for extubation
2. Protect the lung from barotraumas, volutrauma, and infection
3. Improve gas exchange
4. To reduce the work of breathing

Initial Ventilatory Setting for Postoperative Patient

Condition	Mode	Respiratory rate	Tidal volume	PEEP	FiO$_2$	Additional settings	Remark
Airway protection	Assist control SIMV PSV	10–14/min	8 mL/kg	5 cmH$_2$O	100% to start taper to 40%	Peak flow 60 L/min Trigger sensitivity −2 cmH$_2$O	Continue mechanical Ventilator till airway protection is optimal Consider tracheostomy if indicated
Delayed awakening from anesthesia	Assist control SIMV PSV	10–14/min	8–10 mL/kg	5 cmH$_2$O	100% to start taper to 40%	Peak flow 60L/min Trigger sensitivity −2 cmH$_2$O	Wait for the effect of muscle relaxants and sedatives to subside before giving spontaneous breathing trial

CHAPTER 38

Key Points in Ventilating Neuromuscular Diseases

The main problem in the patient with neuromuscular disease (**NMD**) is **respiratory muscle weakness**. These patients usually have **normal respiratory drive** and **normal lungs**.

In NMD, **ventilatory failure** is due to diseases that **impair transmission** of neural input from the **respiratory center** to the **respiratory muscles** or due to conditions that **prevent proper contraction of respiratory muscles**. Typically, the respiratory center itself is unaffected and initiates a normal respiratory drive.

Respiratory muscle weakness gives rise to following changes:
1. Reduced lung volumes and capacity
2. Increased work of breathing
3. Abnormal breathing during sleep
4. Reduction in ability to cough reflected by decreased peak expiratory flow rates
5. Abnormal regulation of breathing

SIGNS AND SYMPTOMS OF PROGRESSIVE NEUROMUSCULAR RESPIRATORY FAILURE

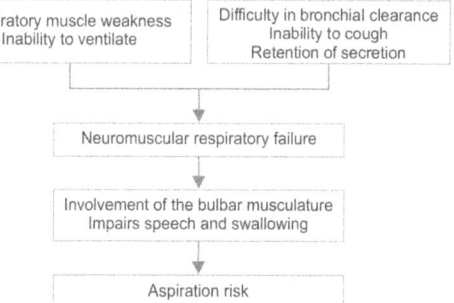

Most common neuromuscular diseases encountered in ICU setting are Guillain–Barré (**GB**) syndrome and **myasthenia gravis**.

Mechanisms underlying acute respiratory failure in myasthenia gravis and GB syndrome	
Upper airway compromise	Both disorders are associated with **weakness** of facial, oropharyngeal, and laryngeal muscles which leads to **mechanical obstruction** of upper airways
	It **interferes** with swallowing, difficulty in maintaining the airway and increased **risk** of aspiration
Weakness of muscles of inspiration	**Weakness** of diaphragm, intercostal muscles, and accessory muscles lead to **inadequate expansion** of lungs with microatelectasis and **compensatory tachycardia**
Weakness of expiratory muscles	**Inadequate cough** and **clearance of secretions** with increased **risk** of aspiration pneumonia
Complications of acute illness	Aspiration and secondary bacterial infection, pulmonary thromboembolism

CLINICAL ASSESSMENT

1. Daily **assessment** of facial, oropharyngeal, and laryngeal weakness
2. Testing for **elevation** of head and neck off the bed to tests the power in **trapezius** and **shoulder muscles**
3. Check **muscle power** in all **limbs**
4. Watch for **nocturnal hypoxia**. Poor pulmonary mechanics in supine position results in 50% decrease in vital capacity causing nocturnal fall in oxygen saturation. It also indicates **impending respiratory failure** due to **diaphragmatic weakness**.
5. Daily assessment of **Single Breath Count** (measure of **vital capacity**): After a deep inspiration, hold the breath, and start counting numbers till the next breath. Normally, one should be able to count up to **30–40**.

GOALS OF MECHANICAL VENTILATION IN CHRONIC NEUROMUSCULAR DISEASE

1. To support muscles of respiration to maintain normal alveolar ventilation
2. To maintain pulmonary compliance

Ventilatory Strategy in Neuromuscular Disease

Mode	Assist control mode, **until** there are signs of clinical recovery
	If **weaning trial** (on **spontaneous mode**) is given, keep **overnight** on assist/control mode to allow **adequate rest** prior to subsequent weaning attempt
Tidal volume	8–10 mL/kg
Flow trigger	**Minimum** to **avoid fatigability**
Positive end-expiratory pressure	Neuromuscular weaknesses are expected to have **reduced** functional residual capacity (**FRC**) and dependent alveolar unit **fails to open** during inspiration
	PEEP has the **beneficial effect** of **reversing** dependent alveolar collapse and helps to **open dependent alveolar** unit during inspiration, hence improve oxygenation

ROLE OF NONINVASIVE VENTILATION

Noninvasive ventilation is an accepted form of respiratory support in patients with NMDs and chest wall disorders provided:

- **Spontaneous** breathing effort is present.
- **Periodic monitoring** of upper airway function/cough reflex/swallowing is performed.
- Serial **blood gas monitoring** is feasible.

Noninvasive Ventilation Settings in Neuromuscular Disease

Mode	BiPAP Biphasic positive airway pressure
IPAP Inspiratory positive airway pressure	8–12 cmH$_2$O
EPAP Expiratory positive airway pressure	3–4 cm H$_2$O
Backup rate	10–12 breaths/min
Active humidification	

CAUTION DURING INTUBATION

Hemodynamic changes and dysautonomia labile blood pressure, bradycardia, increased hypotensive response to sedatives

Patient can get **fatal hyperkalemia** secondary to use of **succinylcholine**

Intubation Strategy

Intubation strategy includes topical anesthesia, small doses of benzodiazepines, atropine if needed, avoidance of succinylcholine.

Fiberoptic intubation is preferred.

Muscle Relaxants

In myasthenia gravis, there is decrease in **effective acetylcholine receptors** as most are blocked by antibodies against the receptors. This results in decrease in **safety margin of nondepolarizing** muscle relaxants leading to increased sensitivity and prolonged effects. **Short**-acting drugs such as atracurium are **safe**.

Inhaled Anesthetics

Inhaled anesthetics such as **halothane** and **isoflurane** have depressant effect on central respiratory drive and neuromuscular junctions and need to be **avoided**.

Monitoring

These patients need extensive monitoring during intubation.

Weaning

Weaning should be tried only when patients show definite signs of **clinical improvement** and are able to **hold** their **neck** and head off the **bed**.

All other criteria for successful weaning such as **improvement** in background disease, normal neurological status (central and peripheral), normal cardiac functions, normal electrolyte and acid–base status, and normal endocrine function also apply to these patients.

In patients with chronic CO_2 retention, **$PaCO_2$** should be kept **above 45** mm Hg to **avoid alkalosis** and **bicarbonate wasting**, which makes weaning more difficult.

Adequate rest must be ensured in between weaning trials.

Treatment Modalities for Difficult Weaning

- Plasmapheresis
- Immunoglobulins
- Minimum use of steroids
- Use of azathioprine and cyclosporine for steroid sparing effect (in myasthenia gravis) should be considered.

Tracheostomy

Early tracheostomy (7–14 days) is indicated in prolonged mechanical ventilation.

Adjunctive therapy in the form of meticulous pulmonary toileting, chest and limb physiotherapy and **psychological motivation** has an important place in management of these patients.

The minimum necessary requirements for extubation are:
1. **Good recovery** in neurological function
2. Minimum secretions
3. Good **ability** to hold the **neck** and **head** off the bed
4. Tidal volume ≥**5 mL**/kg
5. Maximum inspiratory pressure ≤**25** cmH$_2$O

39. Key Points in Ventilating Head/Brain Injury

GOALS OF VENTILATORY STRATEGY IN HEAD/BRAIN INJURY

Early therapeutic intervention in patients with severe head injury is directed toward **airway control:**

1. Maintain **eucapnia**: Normal partial pressure of carbon dioxide (arterial) ($PaCO_2$) levels and avoiding hypocapnia or hypercapnia
2. Maintaining **adequate oxygenation**: Normal partial pressure of arterial oxygen (PaO_2) levels
3. **Minimizing** intra thoracic pressure
4. **Protect** cerebral perfusion:

$$\textbf{CPP} \text{ (cerebral perfusion pressure)} = \textbf{(MAP)} \text{ mean arterial pressure} - \textbf{(ICP)} \text{ intracranial pressure}$$

INDICATIONS FOR INTUBATION AND MECHANICAL VENTILATION IN HEAD/BRAIN INJURY

- Altered level of consciousness/coma causing inadequate protection of the airway can cause **risk of aspiration**
- Glasgow coma score **<8**

- Neurogenic pulmonary edema
- Repeated seizures
- Hypoxemic respiratory failure may be due to aspiration, pneumonia, atelectasis, pulmonary contusion, and pulmonary embolism
- Anticipated neurological deterioration
- Brainstem dysfunction/intracranial hypertension
- Acute lung injury/acute respiratory distress syndrome (**ALI/ARDS**)
- Mean intracranial pressure >**15** mm Hg

GENERAL PRINCIPLES OF MANAGEMENT

- Preference for **oral** intubation
- **Avoid excessive ventilation:** Eucapnia, **PaCO$_2$**—35-40 mm Hg, **EtCO$_2$** monitoring
- **Control intracranial pressure:** Head end elevation—30°, use of sedation and paralytics
- **Avoid hypoxia:** SpO$_2$ target >**95%**

VENTILATORY STRATEGY

Balanced Ventilatory Strategy

To preserve cerebral perfusion, prevent rise in intracranial pressure and balance with principles of **lung protective ventilation**.

1. **Avoid permissive hypercapnia:** Hypercapnia leads to cerebral vasodilatation and increase in cerebral blood volume and intracranial pressure.
2. **Avoid high tidal volume** ventilation as it can lead to **acute lung injury**.

It is recommended to use **low-tidal volume** with **moderate PEEP** (positive end-expiratory pressure).

3. **Prior to suctioning:**
   a. Provide 100% oxygen breath
   b. Supplement additional sedation
   c. Suctioning should be nontraumatic and brief.
4. **To maintain** CPP of **70** mm Hg and mean arterial pressure of **90** mm Hg:
   a. Secure **arterial line** to achieve invasive blood pressure.
   b. **Preload** to be optimized and use of vasopressors if needed.

Ventilatory Strategy

Control mode or assist control mode	Volume control ventilation (**VCV**) Minimal flow ventilation
Fraction of inspired oxygen (FiO$_2$)	Depending on the patient Start with **1**, then decrease by **10–20%** every **20–30** minutes until safe level, i.e., below **0.6**
Inspiratory flow	**60–70** L/min
Tidal volume	**6–8** mL/kg **Adjust minute ventilation** to keep PaCO$_2$ between **30 and 35** mm Hg
Ventilatory rate	**12–14** breaths/min
Inspiratory:expiratory time (**I:E**)	1.2 **Avoid** inverse ratio ventilation
Positive end-expiratory pressure (**PEEP**)	**5–7** cmH$_2$O

Hemodynamic effects of PEEP on intracranial pressure

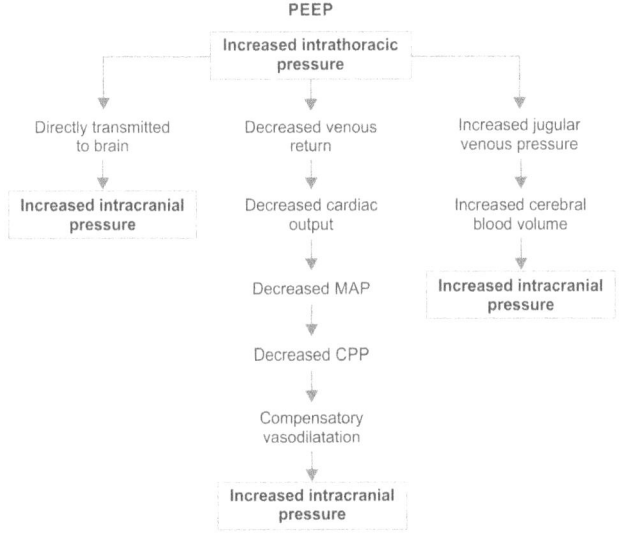

WEANING FROM SEVERE HEAD INJURY

- Normalization of $PaCO_2$ by reduction in ventilatory support
- Complete spontaneous ventilation on T piece or continuous positive airway pressure (CPAP)
- Careful assessment of airway reflexes prior to extubation
- Patient in vegetative state requires tracheostomy

SUMMARY

Traumatic brain injury victims should receive the usual daily care similar to other patients in the intensive care unit.

1. Raising head of bed to **30–45°**; that would **reduce ICP** and **improves CPP**; and **lower** the risk of ventilator associated pneumonia (**VAP**).
2. Keeping the head and neck of the patient in a **neutral** position: this would **improve** cerebral venous drainage and reduce ICP.
3. **Avoiding compression** of **internal** or **external** jugular veins with tight cervical collar or tight tape for fixation of the endotracheal tube that would impede cerebral venous drainage and result in an increase in the ICP.
4. **Turning** the patient **regularly** and frequently with careful observation of the ICP
5. Providing **eye care, mouth,** and **skin** hygiene
6. Implementing all evidence-based bundles for **prevention of infection** including VAP and central line bundle
7. Administrating a **bowel regimen** to **avoid constipation** and **increase of intra-abdominal** pressure and ICP
8. Performing **physiotherapy**

CHAPTER 40: Key Points in Ventilating Severe Asthma

The decision to initiate invasive ventilation in life threatening asthma is made on **clinical grounds**. **Hypercapnia** per say is **not** an indication for intubation as most episodes respond positively to **bronchodilator** therapy and **noninvasive** ventilation. Only **5%** of asthmatic patients need intubation.

INDICATIONS FOR INTUBATION AND VENTILATION

Absolute
- Coma
- Respiratory or cardiac arrest
- Severe refractory hypoxemia

Relative
- **Poor response** to initial management
- Marked **agitation**
- **Depressed** level of **consciousness** with **inability** to protect airway
- Inability to **cooperate** with therapy

- **Silent chest**
  Wheezing and **coarse** airway crepitations may **disappear** as airway obstruction worsens. The silent chest being the sign of **severe airway obstruction**
- Progressive respiratory muscle fatigue and exhausted patient and somnolence
- **Worsening hypoxia** (PaO_2 <60 mm Hg) or cyanosis despite maximal oxygen concentration via face mask (FiO_2 of 60%)
- **Hypercapnia** patient may be having rising $PaCO_2$ with serial blood gas measurements
- Respiratory rate >**35** breaths/min
- Heart rate >**120** beats/min
- Cardiovascular **compromise**

PRECAUTIONS AT THE INITIATION OF VENTILATION

- **Possibility of hypotension**
  It requires optimal preloading with fluids and vasopressors made readily available for use postinduction.
- **Initial hand ventilation** should follow the principles outlined for the mechanical ventilation below and be kept to a **minimum; rate** should be kept **low** and **no PEEP** should be applied.
- **Chest X-ray** should be performed following intubation to assess correct positioning of the endotracheal tube and **exclude pneumothorax**.
- Half of the **life-threatening** complications occur at or around the **time of intubation** in patients

mechanically ventilated for asthma. Intubation should be **smooth** and by **skilled personnel**; repeated manipulation and failed intubation in patients with asthma may prove disastrous.
- Many patients may experience worsening of **severe bronchospasm** if a deeper plane is **not** maintained.

GOALS AND STRATEGY OF MECHANICAL VENTILATION IN SEVERE ASTHMATICS

1. **Controlled hypoventilation:** To **minimize hyperinflation** and to **avoid excessive airway pressures**
2. **Avoid hypoxia** by providing **adequate gas exchange** while **minimizing lung injury**
3. **Early sedation** and **muscle relaxation**
4. Most **important priority is optimization of expiratory time**
5. **Limiting gas trapping**

INITIAL VENTILATOR SETTINGS IN PATIENTS WITH SEVERE ASTHMA

Selection of mode	Assist/control mode
FiO_2	to maintain SaO_2 > 90%
Tidal volume	**4–8** mL/kg (on volume controlled ventilation)
Ventilatory rate	**7–12** breaths/min
Inspiratory time	On pressure controlled ventilation **0.8–1.2** second
Waveform	Decelerating or Square
Extrinsic PEEP	To **offset** 80–90% of auto-PEEP

MONITORING

- Monitor **expired volume** or minute ventilation **(MV)**
- Monitor peak inspiratory pressure/peak pressure (P_{peak}) and plateau pressure $P_{plateau}$
- Blood gas analysis
- **Chest radiographs** in the majority of patients with acute asthma will be **normal** but chest radiographic **examination** is a valuable tool to exclude complications

WEANING

Asthma patients do **not** require ventilatory support for prolonged time. **Settling of bronchospasm** means the asthma attack has resolved in clinical ground, weaning can be attempted. Most can be successfully and easily weaned.

Difficulty in weaning may be in patients with respiratory muscle weakness from hypokalemia, hypophosphatemia, excessive use of **steroids,** and long-term use of **muscle relaxants**.

Chapter 41: Key Points in Ventilating Chronic Obstructive Pulmonary Disease

Clinical manifestations in **exacerbation** of chronic obstructive pulmonary disease (COPD) which become indications for **usage** of mechanical ventilation are:

1. **Hypercapnia**
   High respiratory rate and low-tidal volumes lead to **decreased alveolar ventilation** which leads to **hypoxemia** and CO_2 retention giving rise to **respiratory acidosis**.

2. **Respiratory acidosis**
   Hypercapnia injudicious use of oxygen supplementation leads to **blunting hypoxic** drive of ventilation giving rise to respiratory acidosis.

3. **Intrinsic positive end-expiratory pressure (PEEP)**
   Increased airway resistance leads to prolonged inspiratory time with **inadequate time** for **expiration** which retards **lung emptying**. The reduced lung emptying leads **air trapping**, dynamic hyperinflation, and Intrinsic PEEP.

4. **Respiratory muscle fatigue**
   Intrinsic PEEP leads to augmented inspiratory effort to ventilate the lung which **increases work of breathing** giving rise to respiratory muscle fatigue.

Mechanical ventilation is a challenge in COPD due to following reasons:
1. Disease may **not** have reversible component
2. Bedside **quantification** of COPD is **difficult**
3. **Difficulty to wean** in COPD
4. Steroid-induced **myopathy**
5. **Comorbidities**

GOALS FOR VENTILATOR ASSISTANCE

1. **Relieve** dyspnea and decrease work of breathing
2. Improve **effective** ventilation
3. Improve **arterial blood gas (ABG)**
4. **Buy time** for the precipitating cause of COPD exacerbation to **subside**

Ventilator assistance is provided by **noninvasive** or **invasive** mechanical ventilation.

I. Noninvasive Ventilation

Indications of Noninvasive Ventilation

Tachypnea	RR **>30**/min
	Accessory muscle use and abdominal paradox
ABG	pH **7.2–7.35**
	$PaCO_2$ **>45** mm Hg increase of 10–20 from baseline
PaO_2/FiO_2	**<200** mm Hg
pH	**≤7.30 and/or**
PaO_2	**<60** mm Hg

Provided these values **fail to improve** or **worsen** after trial of **6–8** hours or even earlier) of conservative measure

Avoid noninvasive ventilation (NIV) in COPD if
Patient is **medically unstable,** e.g., cardiogenic or septic shock, acute myocardial infarction with planned intervention, uncontrolled arrhythmia, and uncontrolled upper gastrointestinal bleed.

- Obtunded patient with **poor or irregular** respiratory efforts
- Uncooperative or agitated patient
- Patient **unable to protect** airway
- Patients with **copious** respiratory secretions
- Patients with **recent** upper airway or upper gastrointestinal surgery
- pH **<7.20**, acute rise of $PaCO_2$ **>70** mm Hg
- Unable to get a **correctly fitting mask**
- Patient worsens on NIV or fails to show improvement

Advantages of Treatment with Noninvasive Ventilation

- Prevents intubation
- Decreases mortality
- Facilitates postextubation management
- Less risk of nosocomial intubation

Ventilatory mode—BiPAP is preferred mode

Biphasic Positive Airway Pressure

Inspiratory positive airway pressure (**IPAP**)	12–15 cmH$_2$O to maintain tidal volume 6–7 mL/kg
Expiratory positive airway pressure (**EPAP**)	4–8 cmH$_2$O Increase to improve oxygenation

Weaning Mode

Pressure Support (PS)/CPAP

Pressure Support (**PS**)	**10–15** cmH$_2$O
Continuous positive airway pressure (**CPAP**)	**4–8** cmH$_2$O
Target tidal volume	**6–8** mL/kg
Flow or pressure trigger	to be kept **minimum**
High-flow cycle time	(default ~**25**%) keep ~**40**% in COPD
Rise time	More **gradual**

Pressure support ventilation in COPD patient helps:

1. To reduce respiratory rate
2. To reduce intrinsic PEEP
3. To reduce work of breathing
4. To decrease O$_2$ demand
5. To reduce inspiratory time by manipulating inspiratory flow

II. Intubation and Invasive Mechanical Ventilation

When to Intubate?

1. Worsening of ABG over **1–2** hours or lack of improvement in ABG after **4** hours
2. A **sharp** progressive rise in the **PaCO$_2$** with a **pH <7.2** on **controlled** oxygen therapy
3. **Dangerous hypoxia**, unrelieved on conservative therapy or NPPV
4. Patients showing **poor response** to antibiotics, bronchodilator, and physiotherapy

Goals for ventilator settings:
1. Minimize air trapping
2. Avoid over distension: Plateau pressure <30 cmH$_2$O
3. Provide adequate oxygenation: SpO$_2$ 86-92%
4. Provide adequate ventilation: pH >7.25

Ventilatory Mode: Assist Pressure/Volume Control Mode

Tidal volume:	**6–8** mL/kg reduce tidal volume because the space is reduced in alveoli due to the volume trapped
Ventilatory rate	**8–10** breaths/min
I:E ratio	**1:3** or more (I time of **0.8–1.2 s**)
Flow	**80–90** L/min Faster rise time in pressure control to shorten inspiratory time (provided plateau pressure is not extended beyond **30** cmH$_2$O
Peak inspiratory pressure	up to **50** cmH$_2$O is acceptable PIP is high due to high flow
Plateau pressure	**<30** cmH$_2$O
Trigger sensitivity	Minimal on pressure or flow trigger
Extrinsic PEEP	Start at **3** cmH$_2$O case of any increase in PEEP, look at **peak** inspiratory pressure and **plateau** pressure Any increase in peak inspiratory pressure and plateau pressure, decrease PEEP. Keep a close **watch** on hemodynamics

MONITORING

1. Decrease $PaCO_2$ level to patient's baseline
2. Maintain near normal pH >**7.3**
3. Adequacy of oxygenation
4. Monitor hemodynamic parameters
5. Watch for patient—ventilator asynchrony, excessive pressures, inadequate flows, and volume

KEY POINTS TO REMEMBER

An **elective tracheostomy** is preferred if ventilator support needs to be extended for **>7 days** or the patient has **copious secretions** that cannot be suctioned through the endotracheal tube.

Weaning begins when the **precipitating factor** of the respiratory failure is partially or totally **reversed**.

Factors which **increase resistance** such as size of the endotracheal tube, secretions in the tube, presence of elbow shaped parts, and HME filters in the circuit should be **avoided**.

Dynamic hyperinflation is a **major** determinant of weaning failure.

CHALLENGES IN VENTILATING COPD

- Barotrauma
- Fluid electrolyte and acid-base disturbances
- Pulmonary infections/nosocomial infections
- Arrhythmias precipitated by respiratory acidosis
- Hypotension, right heart failure
- Pneumothorax
- Aspiration
- Weaning difficulty

Key Points in Ventilating Acute Respiratory Distress Syndrome

1. Definition

ARDS new global definition	Classification		
	Mild	**Moderate**	**Severe**
Time of Initiation	Acute onset within **1 week** of a known clinical insult or **New/worsening** respiratory symptoms		
Pulmonary Edema	**Not explained** by intravascular volume **overload** or **Cardiogenic edema**		
Radiological Features	**Bilateral infiltrates** on chest X-ray or CT or lung ultrasound (by trained professional) which is **not** explained by pleural effusion, atelectasis, or nodules		
Hypoxemia	**201–300** with NIV/CPAP	**101–200**	**≤100**
PaO_2/FiO_2	PEEP ≥5 or HFNO >30 L/min	PEEP **≥5**	PEEP **≥5**
Hypoxia SpO_2/FiO_2	<315 with SpO_2 **≤97%**		

Note: ≤: less than equal to/≥: more than equal to

Chapter 42: Key Points in Ventilating Acute Respiratory...

2. Goals of Mechanical Ventilation in Acute Respiratory Distress Syndrome (ARDS)

Maintain **oxygenation**	PaO_2 goal **55–80** mm Hg
Minimize **volutrauma**	Tidal volume (V_T) goal **6 mL/kg** *Ideal body weight (IBW)
Minimize **barotrauma**	Plateau pressure (P_{plat}) **≤30**
Permissive **hypercapnia**	pH **≥7.2**

3. Initial Ventilator Setup

A. Calculate Predicted Body Weight (PBW)

Males	= 50 + 2.3 [height (inches) − 60]
Females	= 45 + 2.3 [height (inches) − 60]

B. Ventilator Mode: Ideal mode: Assist Control Volume Control (**AC–VC**)

C. Tidal Volume (V_T) 6 cc/kg (IBW)

Ideal Body Weight (IBW) Table for V_T 6cc/kg

	Height (inches)	5'0"	5'1"	5'2"	5'3"	5'4"	5'5"	5'6"	5'7"
Tidal Volume (mL)	Male	300	310	330	340	360	370	380	400
	Female	270	290	300	310	330	340	360	370

	Height (inches)	5'8"	5'9"	5'10"	5'11"	6'0"	6'1"	6'2"	6'3"
Tidal Volume (mL)	Male	410	420	440	450	470	480	490	510
	Female	380	400	410	420	440	450	470	480

D. Other Settings

Respiratory Rate (RR): Set initial rate to approximate baseline minute ventilation (not **>35** breaths/min).

FiO₂: 100%
PEEP: Use a minimum PEEP of 5 cmH₂O

4. Ventilator Adjustments in ARDS

Step 1:
Ensure you are meeting your oxygenation goals (PaO₂, 55–80 mm Hg, or SpO₂ 88–96%)

Use of **incremental FiO₂/PEEP** combinations such as shown below can be beneficial in achieving oxygenation goal.

Lower PEEP/higher FiO₂

FiO₂	PEEP
0.3	5
0.4	5
0.4	8
0.5	8
0.5	10
0.6	10
0.7	10
0.7	12
0.7	14
0.8	14
0.9	14
0.9	16
0.9	18
1	18–24

Higher PEEP/lower FiO₂

FiO₂	PEEP
0.3	5
0.3	8
0.3	10
0.3	12
0.3	14
0.4	14
0.4	16
0.5	16
0.5	18
0.5–0.8	20
0.8	22
0.9	22
1	22
1	24

Ensure Ventilator Synchrony
- **Assess sedation requirements**
  Initially include **analgesic + sedation**, later can **switch** to analgesia alone if not paralyzed.
- Goal **sedation score** of **Richmond analgesia and sedation score (RASS) −2 to −3 initially**, target **0-1** once improving (**refer table**)

Richmond Analgesia and Sedation Score

Score		Description
4	Combative	Violent, immediate **danger** to staff
3	Very Agitated	Pulls at or removes tubes, **aggressive**
2	Agitated	Frequent **non purposeful** movement, fights ventilator
1	Restless	Anxious, apprehensive but movements **not aggressive** or vigorous
0	Alert and calm	
−1	Drowsy	Not fully alert, sustained awakening to voice (eye opening and contact **>10** seconds)
−2	Light sedation	Briefly awakens to voice (eye opening and contact **<10** seconds)
−3	Moderate sedation	Movements or eye opening to voice (**no eye** contact)
−4	Deep sedation	**No response** to voice, but movement or eye opening to physical stimulation
−5	Unarousable	**No response** to voice or physical stimulation

> **Step 2:**
> **Perform an inspiratory pause to check the plateau pressure P$_{plat}$ (goal <30)**

Plateau pressure goal: ≤30 cmH$_2$O

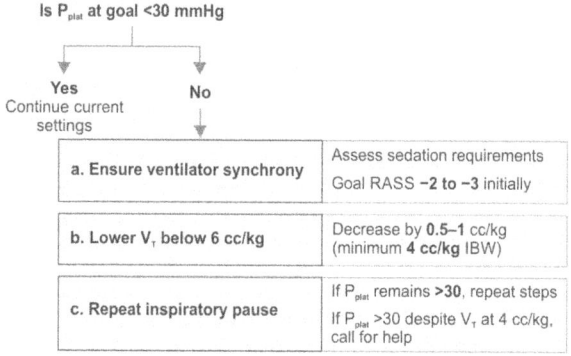

Driving Pressure Titration for PEEP
Driving pressure = P$_{plat}$ − PEEP

Goal is to find **PEEP** that **minimizes Driving pressure**

Step 1: Measure **P$_{plat}$** with **inspiratory pause** of **0.5 seconds**

Step 2: Increase PEEP by **2–4**

Step 3: After **20 seconds** remeasure P$_{plat}$

Step 4: If decrease in driving pressure, **repeat steps 1–3**. If increased or hypotension, return to prior PEEP

	Step 3:
	Check Blood Gas 15–20 minutes after changes to assess adequacy of ventilation

If pH < 7.2	Increase RR, **monitor** for auto-PEEP (intrinsic positive end-expiratory pressure) Consider increasing V_T by **0.5–1** cc/kg, call for help
If pH 7.2–7.40	No changes, permissive hypercapnia **OK** to allow for **low V_T**
If pH > 7.40	Reduce set RR, assess for analgesia/sedation needs

Step 4: Reassess to ensure achieving ARDS ventilation goals

- PaO_2 60–80 mm Hg, SpO_2 (90–94%), V_T (6 cc/kg), P_{plat} (7.2)
- Titrate down FiO_2 for PaO_2 60–80 mm Hg, SpO_2 90–94%

Refractory Hypoxemia

1. **Prone Positioning**
   Provides mortality benefit for **moderate-to-severe** ARDS (**PaO_2:FiO_2 <150**)
   Caution if:
   - Hemodynamic instability
   - Facial/pelvic fractures
   - Arrhythmias

   Prone for at least **16 hours**
   Turn **supine for 4–8 hours**, then reassess candidacy for proning

Repeat steps 2-3 if $PaO_2:FiO_2$ remains **<150 after 4 hours** supine

2. **Neuromuscular Blockade**
   Ensure **adequate sedation (RASS <-4)** before staring paralytic either **bolus** dosing or **bolus followed by infusion**. One may use **cisatracurium** dosing **0.1-0.2** mg/kg bolus, followed by **infusion** dose of **2-10 µ/kg/min**. It is ideal to derive TOF (train of four) to assess adequacy of paralysis. It is noteworthy that paralysis is **NOT** necessary for proning.

3. **Recruitment maneuvers**
   Not routinely recommended
   Set PEEP to 30 for 30 seconds **("30 for 30")** or **"40 for 40"**

4. **Extracorporeal membrane oxygenation**
   In a center equipped with ECMO, call ECMO team if **PaO_2 <80** on **FiO_2 100%** despite proning with hemodynamic instability for 12 hours
   Exclusion criteria: BMI > 45, age >65, >30 pack year smoking history

Key Points to Note
- Plan for **line placement** on **same side** for **safer proning**
- Steroids **NOT** recommended for ARDS management **unless** concomitant refractory septic shock
- **Conservative fluid strategy** and/or **diuresis for negative 24 hours fluid** balance, even if requiring **low dose vasopressors**

CHAPTER 43

Key Points in Care of Patients on Long-term Mechanical Ventilator

1. Shift to **isolation room** if possible/required
2. Use of humidification chamber/heat moisture exchanger in breathing circuit
3. Use of alpha bed, air mattress, and sequential compression device
4. Regular **change of position**, back care to be given
5. Start **enteral feeding** if **not** contraindicated
6. **Analgesia** and **sedation** as required, muscle relaxant only if indicated. Patient may require physical restraint after taking consent from family
7. **Change of intravenous (IV) lines** and extension tubing as per protocol. **Secure central lines** and tubings and ensure correct position
8. **Proper record** of vital parameters and sequence of events
9. Orderly **maintenance** of laboratory reports
10. **Extubation** as per protocol
11. **Tracheostomy** as and when indicated
12. Regular mouth care with **0.12% chlorhexidine** solution

13. Change of wound **dressing**, tracheostomy dressing (if present)
14. Regular oral/endotracheal **suctioning** under strict asepsis
15. Encourage chest and limb **physiotherapy**. Monitor air entry/chest rise, presence of secretions
16. Ascertain optimal **ventilation** and **oxygenation** by monitoring SpO_2, arterial blood gas, and periodic chest X-ray.

CHAPTER 44: Ventilator Troubleshooting

1. Upon hearing any alarm on ventilator—**observe the patient first**, especially in event of disconnection from ventilator
2. **Never ignore** an alarm, or **mute** the alarm without rectifying the issue
3. **Monitor information found on control panel namely:**
   Mode of ventilator
   Tidal volume
   Set frequency of breaths
   FiO_2
   Inspiratory time: Expiratory time ratio (I:E ratio)
   Level of pressure support
   Level of PEEP
   Trigger sensitivity
4. **Monitor the following information found on display panel**
   Peak airway pressure
   Plateau pressure
   Mean airway pressure
   Spontaneous respiratory rate, tidal volume
   Exhaled tidal volume

	Alarm	Cause	Troubleshooting
1.	**Apnea alarm** **especially on PSV/CPAP mode**	**No** breath was delivered or **No** breath was triggered for a period of **apnea** time **pre-set** by operator **Trigger** level setting **inappropriate**	Ensure **sedation** is **omitted,** switch to assist control mode (**ACM**) and re-schedule spontaneous breathing trial (**SBT**) Set **trigger** level appropriately
2.	**High pressure alarm**	**The measured peak inspiratory pressure is higher than the set maximum level due to**	
		Secretions in airway	Suctioning
		Partially blocked endotracheal tube	May even require tube change
		Tube kinking	Release tubing
		Water in the tube	Drain tube
		Biting	Bite block insertion
		Patient-ventilator dyssynchrony	Ensure adequate sedation of patient Reassure patient
		Endobronchial tube	Reposition endotracheal tube
		Coughing	Sedation
		Increased airway resistance	Treat the cause
		Bronchospasm	Bronchodilator

Contd...

Contd…

	Alarm	Cause	Troubleshooting
		Decreased lung compliance	Adjustment of tidal volume and rate to ensure plateau pressure below 28 cmH$_2$O
		Atelectasis	Mucolytics, chest physiotherapy, postural drainage, and bronchoscopic intervention
		Fluid overload	Diuretics, fluid restriction
		Pneumothorax	Immediate intervention/intercostal drain insertion
3.	**Low minute ventilation alarm** **Or**	The measured peak Inspiratory pressure (**PIP**) is **lower** than the set **minimum** level due to **Leak** in circuit or **disconnection**	Check circuit junctions—**tighten**
	Low pressure alarm	Endotracheal tube/tracheostomy tube cuff **deflated**	**Re-inflate**, periodic checking of endotracheal cuff pressure using cuff manometer. **Replace** tube if noted to be having spontaneously deflating cuff

Contd…

Contd...

Alarm		Cause	Troubleshooting
	Or	Endotracheal tube **malposition/ displacement**	Check endotracheal tube **position**
	Low-exhaled volume alarm	**Inadequate** flow	Patient may be requiring higher flow
		Patient **tired** on weaning mode	Change mode, **escalate** pressure support
		Disconnection	**Reconnect** ventilator
4.	**Low SpO$_2$**		Adjust **PEEP** and **FiO$_2$** **Disconnect** patient from ventilator and **manually** ventilate using Bains circuit or AMBU
		Pulse oximeter tracing distorted	**Reattach** pulse oximeter probe
			Auscultation and ensure bilateral air entry Check tube **position** at lip Consider **suctioning** **ABG, chest X-ray** to be obtained
5.	**Air/oxygen blender alarm**	Supply pressure inadequacy	Gas hose fittings to be checked/reinserted into the wall outlets Ensure that wall outlets have adequate pressure

CHAPTER 45: Weaning Criteria

CLINICAL PARAMETERS
- Resolution/stabilization of disease process
- Conscious and alert
- Hemodynamically stable
- Intact cough/gag reflex
- Spontaneous respiration
- Peripheral temperature acceptable
- Adequate urine output
- Acid–base status and electrolytes normal
- All equipment required for reintubation are readily available

Numerical Parameters

Parameters	Normal range	Weaning threshold
PaO_2/FiO_2	>400	>200
Tidal volume	5–7 mL/kg	>5 mL/kg
Respiratory rate	14–18 breaths/min	<40 breaths/min
Vital capacity	65–75 mL/kg	>10 mL/kg
Minute ventilation	5–7 L/min	<10 L/min
Negative inspiratory force	>90 cmH_2O	>25 cmH_2O
Rapid shallow breathing index (f/V_T)	<50	<105

WEANING PROCESS

Explain the process to the patient and encourage cooperation

Begin during daytime, allow patient to **rest at night** and between trials of weaning

Place patient in **propped up** position

Breathe independently for **30 – 120** minutes

Arterial blood gas obtained at end of spontaneous breathing trial

PEEP — 5 cmH$_2$O,
Pressure support (**PS**) 0 – 5 cmH$_2$O
FiO$_2$ <0.5

CRITERIA FOR DISCONTINUATION OF A WEANING TRIAL

1. Tachypnea (**respiratory rate** >35 breaths/min for ≥5 min)
2. Hypoxemia (oxygen saturation by pulse oximeter **<90%**)
3. Tachycardia (heart rate >**140** beats/min or sustained rate increase >**20%**)
4. Bradycardia (sustained rate decrease by >**20%**)
5. Hypertension (systolic BP >**180** mm Hg)
6. Hypotension (systolic BP <**90** mm Hg)
7. Agitation, diaphoresis, anxiety, and respiratory distress (use of **accessory muscles**, **abdominal paradox.**)
8. Optional ABG criteria : Increase in PaCO$_2$ >**10 mmHg** or decrease in **pH >0.1**

Extubation
1. Control of airway reflexes
2. Patent upper airway (air leak around tube)
3. Minimal oxygen requirement
4. Minimal rate
5. Minimize pressure support (0-10 cmH$_2$O)
6. "Awake" patient

SECTION 8

Blood Transfusion

46. Protocol for Blood Transfusion in ICU
47. Protocol for Massive Blood Transfusion

46. Protocol for Blood Transfusion in ICU

The World Health Organization (WHO) recommends safe and rational use of blood and blood products to reduce practices of **unsafe** and **unnecessary transfusions** and to improve safety and outcome in patients. Rational use minimizes adverse events related to transfusion including **technical errors, transfusion reactions,** and **risk of infection transmission.**

Hence blood transfusion should be given when potential clinical **benefits outweigh** the **potential risks** to the patients.

I. Packed Red Blood Cells

Transfusion trigger/indications:

Hemoglobin: <7 g/dL in healthy individual
<8–9 g/dL in cardiovascular disease, elderly, mechanical ventilation, and postchemotherapy.

Dosage: 4 mL/kg

One unit has an average of **300 mL**, will **raise** hemoglobin by **0.8–1 g/dL**

Special instructions to be given if the following RBC products are indicated namely:
- Gamma-irradiated
- Washed RBCs
- Leukoreduced RBCs

II. Platelet Concentrates

Common Causes of Thrombocytopenia in ICU

- Drug induced—heparin, H_2 receptor blockers, Glycoprotein IIb/IIIa **(gp2b3a) inhibitors**, antibiotics such as Linezolid
- Sepsis
- Massive bleeding
- Thrombocytopenia with thrombocytopenic thrombotic purpura (**TTP**), hemolytic uremic syndrome (**HUS**), and disseminated intravascular coagulation (**DIC**)

Indications

- Platelet counts **<10,000/µL** to prevent spontaneous bleeding, and **<20,000/µL** in presence of risk factors of spontaneous bleeding
- Prior to invasive procedures
    maintain **20,000 – 50,000/µL**
- Ophthalmic/neurosurgery
    maintain **>1,00,000/µL**
- Massive transfusion
    maintain **>50,000/µL**

Dosage

- **One unit** of **random** donor platelet (**RDP**) concentrate increases platelet count by **2,000 – 4,000 cells/mm^3**
- **One unit of single** donor platelet is equivalent to giving roughly **six RDPs**
- Transfuse over **30–60 minutes**
- **RhD negative females** in child-bearing age must be given **RhD negative platelets** to **prevent Rh sensitization**

III. Fresh Frozen Plasma
Indications in ICU
- DIC
- Factor deficiency
- Massive transfusion
- INR raised
- Reversal of effect of anticoagulants

Dosage
10–15 mL/kg increases **fibrinogen** level by **1 g/L**.

IV. Cryoprecipitate
Indications
DIC, fibrinogen level <1 g/L, massive transfusion with hypofibrinogenemia.

Dosage
Standard **adult dose** of cryoprecipitate (**3–4 g fibrinogen**) is equivalent to **10 bags** of whole blood cryoprecipitate would **raise** the plasma fibrinogen by **1 g/L**.

General Protocol

1. Sample for blood grouping and crossmatching should be withdrawn after correctly identifying patient requiring transfusion. Sample must be drawn from either **peripheral vein** or **central venous access** in **EDTA bulb** and should be correctly labeled.
2. **Requisition form** should be filled correctly by registered medical practitioner and signed. Details on the form include:
    - Patients demographic data
    - Diagnosis
    - Indication of blood transfusion
    - **Quantity of blood** and **blood components** to be **reserved** including packed red blood cells (PRBCs), fresh frozen plasma, platelet component (single donor or random donor), cryoprecipitate
    - Details of past blood transfusion
    - History of adverse blood transfusion reaction
3. Required quantity of blood products should be issued when indicated.
4. Correctly identify recipient prior to starting transfusion.
5. **Meticulous checking** of the issued blood should be done and documented, including patient name, blood group, donor's blood group,

unit number of the blood product, date of collection and expiry.

6. Start transfusion within a **maximum of 30 minutes** after issue from the blood bank. Blood should not be routinely warmed. Premedication of diuretic or antihistaminic should be given only when indicated.

Blood and Blood Component Flow Rates in Non Emergent Scenario

Blood component	Flow rate initial 15 minutes	Flow rate after 15 minutes
Packed red blood cells	60–120 mL/h	4 mL/min or 240 mL/h
Fresh frozen plasma	2–5 mL/min 120–300 mL/h	300 mL/h or as tolerated
Platelet concentrate	2–5 mL/min 120–300 mL/h	300 mL/h or as tolerated
Cryoprecipitate	Rapid infusion	

7. **Blood administration sets** (with **170 mm filter**) are to be used for all blood components and change blood sets **after 4 hours** due to likelihood of **bacterial contamination**. To use leukocyte depletion filter when indicated.

8. Patient's **vitals** should be monitored during the period of transfusion and documented.

9. **Flush IV line** with **normal saline**. Do **NOT** routinely coadminister any other IV fluid

through the same line used for blood components (especially Ringer's lactate and 5% dextrose).

10. Massive transfusion protocol to be **activated** in following situations:
    - Loss of one blood volume within a 24 hours period
    - Loss of 50% of blood volume within 3 hours
    - Loss of blood at rate in excess of 150 mL/min

11. **In case of adverse transfusion reaction**
    - **Stop transfusion** immediately, keep **IV line open with normal saline**
    - Counter check blood bag, crossmatching report, and patient identity
    - Notify blood bank
    - Collect venous blood sample from a vein on arm opposite to site of intravenous access used for transfusion and send it in **EDTA bulb** to blood bank along with the blood bag, blood transfusion set, and first voided urine sample
    - Monitor patient, manage airway breathing and circulation, antihistamine, antipyretic, and steroid if indicated

12. Empty plastic blood containers, needles, and tubings should be discarded as per **biomedical waste disposal** instructions.

CHAPTER 47

Protocol for Massive Blood Transfusion

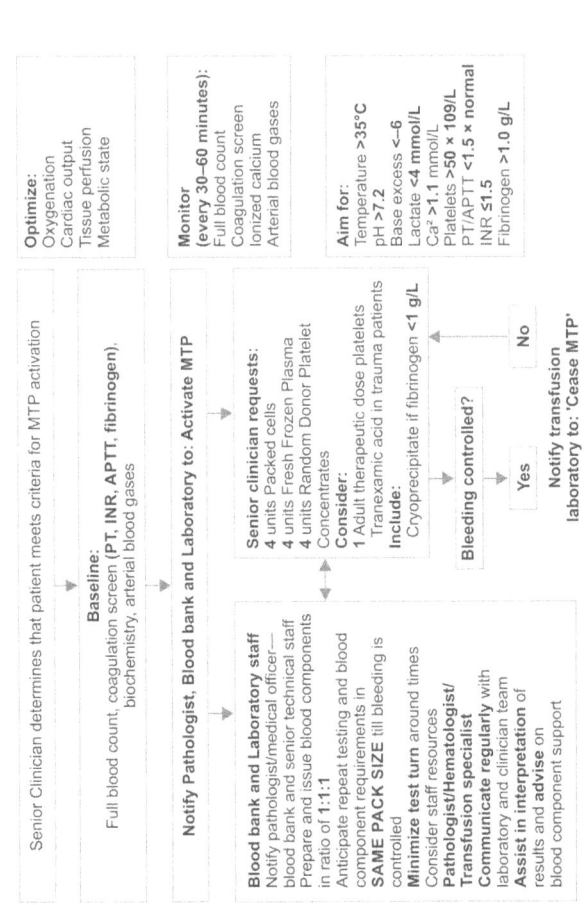

SECTION 9: Scoring System in ICU

48. SOFA Score
49. Child Pugh Score for Liver Disease
50. Clinical Pulmonary Infection Score for Ventilator Associated Pneumonia
51. Wells Score for Predicting Risk of Pulmonary Embolism (PE)
52. Pulmonary Embolism Severity Index (PESI) Score
53. Acute Physiological and Chronic Health Evaluation (APACHE)-II Score
54. Score for Atrial Fibrillation Stroke Risk: CHA_2DS_2VASc

CHAPTER 48: SOFA Score

SOFA score	0	1	2	3	4
Respiratory: PaO_2/FiO_2	>400	<400	<300	<200	<100
Cardiovascular: Doses of vasopressors in µg/kg/min	No Hypotension / MAP >70 mm Hg	MAP <70 mm Hg	Dopamine <5 or Dobutamine (any dose)	Dopamine 5.1–15 or Epinephrine ≤0.1 or Norepinephrine ≤0.1	Dopamine >15 or Epinephrine >0.1 or Norepinephrine >0.1
Central nervous system: GCS	15	13–15	10–12	6–9	<6
Liver: Bilirubin (mg/dL)	<1.2	1.2–1.9	2–5.9	6–11.9	>12
Coagulation: Platelet count ($10^3/\mu L$)	>150	<150	<100	<50	<20
Renal: Creatinine mg/dL/urine output	<1.2	1.2–1.9	2–3.4	3.5–4.9/<500 mL	>5/<200 mL

Score	Mortality
0–6	<2%
7–9	0–10%
10–12	10–30%
13–14	40–60%
15	75–90%
16–24	>90%

CHAPTER 49

Child Pugh Score for Liver Disease

Child Pugh Score for liver disease	1	2	3
Ascites	Absent	Slight	Moderate
Bilirubin (mg/dL)	<2	2–3	>3
Albumin (g/dL)	>3.5	2.8–3.5	<2.8
Prothrombin time (second over control) or INR	<4/<1.7	4–6 /1.7–2.3	>6/>2.3
Encephalopathy	None	Grade 1–2 Mild to moderate	Grade 3–4 Severe

	Class A	Class B	Class C
Total points	5–6	7–9	10–15
1 year survival	100%	80%	45%

Chapter 50: Clinical Pulmonary Infection Score for Ventilator Associated Pneumonia

Clinical pulmonary infection score	0	1	2
Tracheal secretions	Rare	Abundant	Abundant + Purulent
Chest X-ray infiltrates	No infiltrate	Diffused	Localized
Temperature (°C)	≥36.5 and ≤38.4	≥38.5 and ≤38.9	≥39 or ≤36
Leukocyte count (per mm^3)	≥4,000 and ≤11,000	<4,000 or >11,000	<4,000 or >11,000 + band forms ≥500
PaO$_2$/FiO$_2$ ratio	>240 or ARDS		≤240 and no evidence of ARDS
Microbiology/Culture	Negative		Positive

Score >6 is suggestive of pneumonia

CHAPTER 51
Wells Score for Predicting Risk of Pulmonary Embolism (PE)

Criteria	Points
Clinical signs and symptoms of deep vein thrombosis	3
Pulmonary embolism is most likely diagnosis	3
Tachycardia (heart rate >100/min)	1.5
Immobilization/surgery in last 4 weeks	1.5
Prior deep vein thrombosis or pulmonary embolism	1.5
Hemoptysis	1
Active malignancy	1

Points	Risk
<2	Low
2–6	Intermediate
>6	High

Points	Likelihood of PE
0–4	Unlikely
>4	Likely

CHAPTER 52

Pulmonary Embolism Severity Index (PESI) Score

Predictor	Points
Age	1 point/year
Male sex	10
Cancer	30
Heart failure	10
Chronic lung disease	10
Pulse ≥110/min	20
Systolic blood pressure <100 mm Hg	30
Respiratory rate ≥20/min	20
Temperature <36°C	20
Altered mental status	60
Arterial oxygen saturation <90%	20

Class	Score	30-day mortality
I	<65	1.10%
II	66–85	3.10%
III	86–105	6.50%
IV	106–125	10.40%
V	>125	24.50%

CHAPTER 53

Acute Physiological and Chronic Health Evaluation (APACHE)-II Score

APACHE Score	High abnormal range			Normal	Low abnormal range			
A = Acute Physiologic Score	4	3	2	1	0	1	2	3	4

	4	3	2	1	0	1	2	3	4
Physiological variables									
Rectal temperature (°C)	≥41	39–40.9		38.5–38.9	36–38.4	34–35.9	32–33.9	30–31.9	≤29.9
MAP	≥160	130–159	110–129		70–109		50–69		≤49
Heart rate	≥180	140–179	110–139		70–109			40–54	≤39
Respiratory rate	≥50	35–49		25–34	12–24				≤5
A-a DO_2 (FiO_2 ≥0.5)	≥500	350–499	200–349		<200				
PaO_2 (FiO_2 <0.5)					>70	61–70		55–60	<55
Arterial pH	>7.7	7.6–7.69		7.5–7.59	7.33–7.49		7.25–7.32	7.15–7.24	<7.15
HCO_3	≥52	41–51.9		32–40.9	22–31.9		1–21.9	15–17.9	<15
Potassium	≥7	6–6.9		5.5–5.9	3.5–5.4	3–3.4	2.5–2.9		<2.5
Sodium	≥180	160–179	155–159	150–154	130–149		120–129	111–119	≤110
Creatinine	≥3.5	2–3.4	1.5–1.9		0.6–1.4		<0.6		
Hematocrit	≥60		50–59.9	46–49.9	30–45.9		20–29.9		<20
WBC	≥40		20–39.9	15–19.9	3–14.9		1.2–9		<1
GCS					Score = GCS – 15				

B = Age points Age score

Age	Score
≤44	0
45–54	2
55–64	3
65–74	5
≥75	6

C = Chronic health points

Chronic health insufficiency	Score
Nonoperative	5
Emergent operative	5
Elective operative	2

APACHE score = A + B + C

Score	Predicted mortality rate
0–4	4%
5–9	8%
10–14	15%
15–19	25%
20–24	40%
25–29	55%
30–34	75%
35 and above	85%

Chapter 54: Score for Atrial Fibrillation Stroke Risk: CHA$_2$DS$_2$VASc

Risk	Score
Congestive heart failure/left ventricular dysfunction	1
Hypertension	1
Age ≥75 years	2
Diabetes mellitus	1
Stroke/transient ischemic attack	2
Vascular disease (prior myocardia; infarction, peripheral arterial disease, aortic plaque)	1
Age 65–74 years	1
Female	1

Total score	Risk of stroke	
0	0.20%	Low
1	0.60%	Moderate
2	2.20%	High
3	3.20%	
4	4.80%	
5	7.20%	
6	9.70%	
7	11.20%	
8	10.80%	
9	12.20%	

Score
0 = **No therapy recommended**
1 = **Aspirin or oral anticoagulant should be considered**
≥2 = **Oral anticoagulant is recommended**

Section 10: Bedside Hemodialysis in ICU

55. Protocol for Dialysis

Chapter 55: Protocol for Dialysis

Priming Procedure

1.	Switch **ON** the machine
2.	Start **HOT** rinse
3.	Pass preliminary (T_1) test
4.	Attach dialyzer and blood tubing to machine
5.	Connect normal saline with IV set
6.	Attach Hanson connector to dialyzer
7.	**FLUSH** all monitor lines with normal saline **1 L**
8.	Remove all air
9.	Start recirculation
10.	Recheck if any air is present and remove it
11.	Flush all monitor lines with **NORMAL SALINE**
12.	Start dialysis

Intradialysis Patient Monitoring

Monitor **patient's vital signs** (BP, pulse, SpO$_2$, and RBSL) **and document them**	
Monitor **machines parameters and document** them in Dialysis Chart	
Venous pressure **(VP)**	Ultrafiltration achieved **(UF achieved)**
Arterial pressure **(AP)**	Blood flow rate **(BFR)**
Transmembranous pressure **(TMP)**	Conductivity
Ultrafiltration rate **(UFR)**	Blood sugar level **(BSL)**

Termination Procedure

1.	Check blood pressure and pulse
2.	Check if any blood sample is to be collected
3.	Check if any medicines must be given post-HD
4.	Attach connector to IV set
5.	Take **20 mL NS** in syringe for flushing catheter
6.	Stop blood pump, disconnect arterial line
7.	Connect arterial line with connector and NS
8.	Reinfuse blood back to patient
9.	Disconnect venous line
10.	Give **HEPARIN Lock** to catheter
11.	Remove dialyzer and blood tubing from machine
12.	Start **HOT** disinfection

Maintenance of Dialysis Machine

Program		Frequency
Hot rinse		**Every** day
Hot disinfection	1	After dialysis
	2	If **NO** dialysis, then every **48** hours
Cleaning **Front** supply		**Every** weekly
Surface cleaning	1	Before dialysis
	2	After dialysis
Dialysis Fluid Filter Changing		**90** days or **100** dialysis whichever comes earlier

SECTION 11

Documentation and Checklists

56. Protocol for Intubation Trolley
57. Protocol for Making Sterile Sets
58. Transfer out/Death Report
59. Protocol to Write Death Report

CHAPTER 56: Protocol for Intubation Trolley

Items	Sizes						No.
Face Mask	2	3	4				1 each
Laryngoscope with blades	2	3	4				1 each
Endotracheal tubes	4	4.5	5	5.5			3 each
	6	6.5	7	7.5	8	8.5	4 each
Tracheostomy tubes	7	8					1 each
IV cannula plasters	10						1 each
ETT tie and plasters							4 each
Oropharyngeal airways	2	3	4				1 each
Stylet							1 each
Bougie							1 each
Magill's forceps							1 each
Bain's circuit							1 each
Ambu bag							1 each
Gloves	7	7.5					2 each
O_2 mask with nebuliser and tubing							1 each
T-piece with nebuliser and tubing							1 each
Lignocaine jelly							1 each
Suction catheter	12 F						4 each

Contd...

Contd...

Items	Sizes			No.
Dressing pads/cotton				6 No.
Spirit				1 bottle
Needles	20 G	21 G		10 each
IV cannulae	18 G			3 each
	20 G			3 each
	22 G			3 each
Three ways				3 each
Chest leads				2 Sets
Syringes	2 CC			3 each
	5 CC			3 each
	10 CC			3 each
Scissors				1 each
Blade				2 each
Ryle's tube	16 F	14 F		1 each
IV sets				2 each
Normal saline 100 mL				1 bottle
IV Lignocaine (Xylocard)	4%			1 each
Lignocaine vial	2%	4%		1 each
Injection Adrenaline				2 each

CHAPTER 57

Protocol for Making Sterile Sets

LP set	
Steel bowl	1
Sponge holder	1
Plain bulbs	5
Total instruments	**7**

CVP set	
Sponge holder	1
Steel bowl	1
Plain forceps	1
Needle holder	1
Total instruments	**4**

Bone marrow set	
Sponge holder	1
Steel bowl	1
Bone marrow needle with stylet	1
Total instruments	**3**

Dressing set	
Sponge holder	1
Straight artery forceps	1
Toothed forceps	1
Needle holder	1
With straight artery forceps	1
Total instruments	**5**

ICU tracheostomy set	
Sponge holder	2
Plain forceps	1
Toothed forceps	1
BP handle	1
C-shape retractor	1
Single hook	2
Double hook	2
Needle holder	1
Mosquito artery forceps	4
Curved artery forceps	1
Alleys forceps	2
Tracheal dilator	1
Trocar	1
Steel bowl (small)	1
Total instruments	**21**

CHAPTER 58: Transfer Out/Death Report

Name: Age/Sex:
Hospital No.:

Date of Admission: Date of Discharge/Death:
Time of Admission: Time of Discharge/Death
ICU Resident: ICU Resident:

I. History
Date of admission in ward
ICU call sent at
Examination findings including RR and GCS

II. On Admission in ICU
Examination findings including RR and GCS

III. Course in ICU
1. Significant Laboratory findings/ABG at admission
2. Oxygen therapy/Put on NIV or Intubated and put on invasive ventilator
3. Vitals at that time   ABG at that time, if done
4. Issues
   GCS and Nervous system
   CVS: Inotropes +/−   Renal—AKI, CKD, HD
   GIT – Ileus, distension
   Hematological   Biochemical

Contd...

Contd...

    Infections/Cultures/Antibiotics
    Radiological: CXR, USG, CT, MRI
    Other special investigations
    Special procedures performed/Surgical intervention
    Worsened/Improved over? Days
    Ventilated for? Days
    If tracheostomized, on which day?
    Extubation/Reintubation/NIV postextubation
    Blood products and indications
    Specialist opinion
        *ABG to be mentioned on intubation day (Pre and Post) and on extubation/reintubation/NIV postextubation or if any special events

IV. Details at time of shifting to ward (in cases of discharge)

Condition of patient at time of discharge
ABG to be mentioned on discharge
Time at which call was given to ward for transfer out
Actual time when patient was shifted to ward

V. Time of cardiac arrest/Time of declaration of death

Details of diagnosis of death (Protocol to write death)
Time of filling of Death Certificate by concerned unit resident
Cause of death

CHAPTER 59

Protocol to Write Death Report

Duration of CPCR _____ minutes

Pulse, blood pressure—**not** recordable

Carotids—**not** felt

Heart sounds—**not** audible on auscultation

GCS—3/15

Both pupils—dilated and **not** reacting to light

Reversible causes—**ruled out**

Declared dead at _____ on _____.

Sign and Name of the ICU Resident

SECTION 12
Waste Management and Decontamination

60. Anesthetic Assistant or Technician: Decontamination of Environment and Equipments in ICU
61. Nursing Staff: Decontamination of Environment and Equipments in ICU
62. Housekeeping Personnel: Decontamination of Environment and Equipments in ICU
63. ICU Attendant: Decontamination of Environment and Equipments in ICU
64. Waste Disposal

CHAPTER 60

Anesthetic Assistant or Technician: Decontamination of Environment and Equipments in ICU

No.	Items	Cleaning process	Shift 1	Shift 2	Shift 3
1.	BP apparatus	Wipe with **70% alcohol**. Clean between patient use	After each use		
2.	Blood pressure cuff Tourniquets	Clean with cloth soaked in **soap** and **water**, dry thoroughly. If contaminated with blood/body fluids **spray Bacillol**	After each patient		
3.	Laryngoscope and blade	Handle: Wash with **detergent** and **hot water** and dry thoroughly/use **100 mL Clorox in 900 mL of water** solution spray	After each use		
		Blade: Dip in **100 mL Clorox in 900 mL of water** solution for 10 minutes	After each use		
4.	ECG machine and cables	Clean with **70% alcohol** after use	After each use		
5.	X-ray cassette	Damp wipe with **Clorox**	After each use		
6.	Ultrasound machine	Damp wipe with **100 mL Clorox in 900 mL of water**	After each use		X
	Transducers				X
	Handle and cable	**Alcohol swab**			X
7.	Defibrillator	Damp wipe with **Bacillol**			X
8.	Biomedical equipment	Refer to **manufacturer's** instructions	X	X	X

Contd...

Contd...

No.	Items	Cleaning process	Shift 1	Shift 2	Shift 3
9.	Crash cart trolley and intubation trolley	Disinfect with **Bacillol**	X	X	X
10.	Cardiac monitor	Wipe the screen with **alcohol**. Body can be wiped with **Bacillol**. Allow to dry	X	X	X
11.	Glucometer	Damp wipe with **Bacillol**	X	X	X
12.	Ceilings	When visibly soiled, wash with detergent and **water**			

Bacillol® contains **ethanol** and **propranolol**.
Clorox® is commercially available solution containing sodium **hydroxide**, sodium **hypochlorite**, sodium **chloride**, sodium **carbonate**, and sodium **polyacrylate**.

CHAPTER 61

Nursing Staff: Decontamination of Environment and Equipments in ICU

No.	Items	Cleaning process	Staff responsible	Shift 1	Shift 2	Shift 3
1.	Airways/ventilator tubes	Disposable	Nursing staff	After each patient		
2.	Ambu bags	Dip in **Clorox** for **5** minutes	Nursing staff	After each patient and every **72** hours		
3.	Tourniquet	Alcohol swab	Nursing staff	After each use		
4.	Stethoscopes	Clean with **70% alcohol** after use	Nursing staff	X	X	X
5.	Thermometers	Clean with **detergent** and **water**. Wipe with **70%** alcohol. Store dry	Nursing staff	X	X	X
6.	Dressing trolleys	Disinfect with **Bacillol**	Nursing staff		X	X
7.	Scissors	Clean with **detergent** and **water**. Wipe with **70%** alcohol. Store dry	Nursing staff			X

CHAPTER 62

Housekeeping Personnel: Decontamination of Environment and Equipments in ICU

No.	Items	Cleaning process	Staff responsible	Shift 1	Shift 2	Shift 3
1.	Ventilators	Wipe the surfaces of the ventilator clean, working from the top to the bottom	Housekeeping personnel	X		
2.		Wipe the screen with **alcohol**				
3.		Body can be wiped with **Clorox**				
4.		Allow to dry				
5.	Surface cleaning (horizontal surfaces, windowsills, doorknobs, light switches, furniture in nursing station, and racks)	Disinfect with **Clorox** daily and whenever visibly soiled	Housekeeping personnel	X		

Contd...

Contd...

No.	Items	Cleaning process	Staff responsible	Shift 1	Shift 2	Shift 3
6.	Sinks	Scrub with a separate brush with **detergent** and **water**. Disinfect with **1% sodium hypochlorite** (contact time **10** minutes)	Housekeeping personnel	X		
7.	Walls	Wall to be cleaned with **soap** and **warm water**, followed by disinfection with **Clorox**, once a **month** scrubbing of walls with soap and warm water recommended	Housekeeping personnel	X		Spot cleaning only when soiled
8.	Waste emptying	Collect waste from all areas at least daily or more frequently as needed. Avoid overflowing	Housekeeping personnel	X	X	
9.	Suction Jars	Emptied carefully and disinfect with **100 mL Clorox** in **900 mL** of water solution by dipping for **10** minutes	Housekeeping personnel	X	X	
10.	Waste bins	Clean with **detergent** and **water** and disinfect with **1%** sodium hypochlorite solution (contact time **10** minutes)	Housekeeping personnel	X		X

Contd...

Contd...

No.	Items	Cleaning process	Staff responsible	Shift 1	Shift 2	Shift 3
11.	Bed-rails/bed-frames/bedside table/overbed table	Disinfect with **1%** sodium hypochlorite solution	Housekeeping personnel	x	x	x
12.	IV stands	Disinfect with **1%** sodium hypochlorite solution	Housekeeping personnel	x	x	x
13.	Wall-mounted oxygen and suction fixtures	Damp wipe with **Clorox**	Housekeeping personnel	x	x	x
14.	Telephones	Clean with **70%** alcohol	Housekeeping personnel	x	x	x
15.	Soap dispenser	The casing and the nozzle of the soap dispenser should be cleaned daily with **water** and **detergent**. Wipe clean with **1%** sodium hypochlorite solution and let air dry. Do **not** top up liquid soap	Housekeeping personnel	x	x	x

Contd...

Contd...

No.	Items	Cleaning process	Staff responsible	Shift 1	Shift 2	Shift 3
16.	Floors	Wet cleaning and disinfection with hypochlorite	Housekeeping personnel	X	X	X
17.	Commodes and toilet seats	Clean with **detergent** soap and **water**. Keep dry	Housekeeping personnel	X	X	X
18.	Buckets	Clean with water and detergent after use. Disinfect with **1%** sodium hypochlorite solution. Dry and store inverted	Housekeeping personnel	X	X	X
19.	Mops heads	Disinfect with **1%** sodium hypochlorite solution	Housekeeping personnel	X	X	X
20.	Portable X-ray machine	Damp wipe with **Clorox**	Housekeeping personnel			X
21.	Wheelchairs/trolleys	Clean with detergent and water. Disinfect **1%** sodium hypochlorite solution and let air dry	Housekeeping personnel			X
22.	Slippers	Wash with **detergent** and **water** every night	Housekeeping personnel			X

CHAPTER 63

ICU Attendant: Decontamination of Environment and Equipments in ICU

No.	Items	Cleaning process	Staff responsible	Shift 1	Shift 2	Shift 3
1.	Air mattresses, bed mattresses and pillows	Check regularly to ensure the cover is intact. If damaged it must be discarded and changed. The mattress cover should be washed with detergent and water on patient discharge and disinfected with **1%** Sodium hypochlorite solution (contact time **10 minutes**)	ICU attendant	After each patient or when soiled		
2.	Soiled linen	Collect soiled linen in closed, leak proof containers	ICU attendant	X		
3.	Privacy curtains	Should be laundered monthly and when visibly soiled	ICU attendant	X		
4.	Bedpans/urinals	Reusable after wash with soap and water. Immerse in **1%** sodium hypochlorite solution (contact time **30 minutes**)	ICU attendant			X
5.	Bowls (patient)	Clean with detergent and water. Rinse and dry thoroughly. Disinfect with 1% sodium hypochlorite solution let air dry. Store inverted	ICU attendant			X

CHAPTER 64

Waste Disposal

Biomedical waste	General hospital waste	Incinerable	Sharp container
Plastic/Rubber	Plastic wrappers	Soiled cotton/ Gauze pieces	Needles/Surgical blade
Syringes/ Catheters	Paper bags	Pampers contaminated with body fluid	Broken glass items
Gloves/ IV tubings	Plastic bottles		Scalp vein/ Jelco stylet
Tracheostomy	Needle caps	Microbiological waste	Stapler
Urobag/Drain	Ointment tubes/Tins	Pathological waste	Guidewire
Red bin	**Black bin**	**Yellow bin**	
Contaminated waste	**Recycling**	**Contaminated**	

Glossary

A/C or AC	Assist control
A:G	Albumin:globulin
A-a	Alveolar-arterial oxygen gradient
ABG	Arterial blood gas
ACLS	Advanced cardiac life support
ACM	Assist control mode
ADA	Adenosine deaminase
ADH	Antidiuretic hormone
AFB	Acid-fast bacilli
AG	Anion gap
AGc	Corrected anion gap
AKI	Acute kidney injury
ALI	Acute liver injury
ALP	Alkaline phosphatase
AMBU	Artificial manual breathing unit
AP	Arterial pressure
APACHE	Acute physiological and chronic health evaluation
aPTT	Activated prothrombin time
ARDS	Acute respiratory distress syndrome
BFR	Blood flow rate
BG	Blood glucose
BiPAP	Biphasic positive airway pressure
BLBLI	Beta-lactam beta-lactamase inhibitor
BMI	Body mass index

BP	Blood pressure
BSL	Blood sugar level
Ca	Calcium
CAUTI	Catheter-associated urinary tract infection
CBC	Complete blood count
CH	Complete hemogram
CHF	Congestive heart failure
CKD	Chronic kidney disease
Cl	Chloride
CNS	Central nervous system
CO_2	Carbon dioxide
CONS	Coagulase negative *Staphylococcus aureus*
COPD	Chronic obstructive pulmonary disease
CPAP	Continuous positive airway pressure
CPCR	Cardio-pulmonary-cerebral resuscitation
CPK-MB	Creatine phosphokinase-MB
CPP	Cerebral perfusion pressure
CPR	Cardio-pulmonary resuscitation
CRRT	Continuous renal replacement therapy
CSF	Cerebrospinal fluid
CT	Computed tomography
CTPA	Computed tomography pulmonary angiography
CV	Central venous
CVA	Cerebrovascular accident
CVC	Central venous catheter
CVP	Central venous pressure
CVS	Cardiovascular system
CXR	Chest X-ray

DC	Differential count
DIC	Disseminated intravascular coagulation
DNS	Dextrose normal saline
DO_2	Delivery of oxygen
ECF	Extracellular fluid
ECG	Electrocardiogram
ECV	Extracellular volume
EDTA	Ethylenediaminetetraacetic acid
EEG	Electroencephalogram
ELISA	Enzyme-linked immunosorbent assay
EPAP	Expiratory positive airway pressure
ESBL	Extended-spectrum beta-lactam
ESR	Erythrocyte sedimentation rate
$EtCO_2$	End-tidal carbon dioxide
ETT	Endotracheal tube
f	Frequency
f/V_T	Frequency/tidal volume
FDP	Fibrinogen degradation product
FiO_2	Fraction of inspired oxygen
FRC	Functional residual capacity
G	Gauge
GB	Guillain–Barré
GCS	Glasgow Coma Score
GIT	Gastrointestinal tract
H^+	Hydrogen
H_2O	Water
Hb	Hemoglobin
HCO_3	Bicarbonate
Hct	Hematocrit

HD	Hemodialysis
HFNO	High-flow nasal oxygen
HIV	Human immunodeficiency virus
HR	Heart rate
HRCT	High-resolution contrast CT
HSV	Herpes simplex virus
HTN	Hypertension
HUS	Hemolytic uremic syndrome
I:E	Inspiratory:expiratory time
IBW	Ideal body weight
ICP	Intracranial pressure
ICU	Intensive care unit
INR	International standardized ratio
IPAP	Inspiratory positive airway pressure
IPPV	Intermittent positive pressure ventilation
IV	Intravenous
J	Joules
K	Potassium
kcal	Kilo calorie
KCl	Potassium chloride
LFT	Liver function test
LP	Lumbar puncture
MAP	Mean arterial pressure
MDR	Multidrug resistant
Mg	Magnesium
MODS	Multiorgan dysfunction syndrome
mOsm	Milli osmoles
MRI	Magnetic resonance imaging
MRSA	Methicillin-resistant *Staphylococcus aureus*

MTP	Massive transfusion protocol
MV	Minute ventilation
Na	Sodium
NaCl	Sodium chloride
$NaHCO_3$	Sodium bicarbonate
NIPPV	Noninvasive positive pressure ventilation
NIV	Noninvasive ventilation
NMBA	Neuromuscular blocking agent
NMD	Neuromuscular diseases
NPPV	Noninvasive positive pressure ventilation
NS	Normal saline
NSAIDs	Nonsteroidal anti-inflammatory drugs
NTG	Nitroglycerine
O_2	Oxygen
OSF	Organ system failure
PAC	Pulmonary arterial catheter
$PaCO_2$	Partial pressure of carbon dioxide (arterial)
PAD	Peripheral arterial disease
PaO_2	Partial pressure of arterial oxygen
PAO_2	Partial pressure of alveolar oxygen
P_B	Barometric pressure
PBW	Predicted body weight
PCR	Polymerase chain reaction
PCV	Packed cell volume
PEA	Pulseless electrical activity
PEEP	Positive end-expiratory pressure
PESI	Pulmonary embolism severity index
PFT	Pulmonary function test
P_{H_2O}	Partial pressure of water

PiCCO	Pulse index continuous cardiac output
PiO$_2$	Partial pressure of inspired oxygen
PIP	Peak inspiratory pressure
P$_{peak}$	Peak inspiratory pressure
P$_{plat}$	Plateau pressure
PRBC	Packed red blood cells
PS	Pressure support
PSV	Pressure support ventilation
PT	Prothrombin time
R	Respiratory quotient
RASS	Richmond agitation and sedation score
RBCs	Red blood cells
RBSL	Random blood sugar level
RDP	Random donor platelet
RFT	Renal function test
Rh	Rhesus factor
RL	Ringer lactate
ROSC	Return of spontaneous circulation
RR	Respiratory rate
SAH	Subarachnoid hemorrhage
SaO$_2$	Arterial oxygen saturation
SBC	Single breath count
SBP	Systolic blood pressure
SBT	Spontaneous breathing trial
SDP	Single donor platelets
SGOT	Serum glutamic-oxaloacetic transaminase
SGPT	Serum glutamic-pyruvic transaminase
SIADH	Syndrome of insufficient antidiuretic hormone

SIMV	Synchronized intermittent mandatory ventilation
SLED	Sustained low-efficiency dialysis
SMP	Smear for malarial parasite
SOFA	Sequential organ failure assessment
SpO_2	Oxygen saturation on pulse-oximetry
SvO_2	Venous oxygen saturation
T_3	Triiodothyronine
T_4	Thyroxine
TB	Tuberculosis
TBI	Traumatic brain injury
TBW	Total body water
TC	Total count (WBC)
TMP	Transmembrane pressure
TSH	Thyroid-stimulating hormone
TTP	Thrombotic thrombocytopenic purpura
UAG	Urinary anion gap
UF	Ultrafiltrate
UGI	Upper gastrointestinal
Uk	Urinary potassium
UNa	Urinary sodium
UOP	Urine output
Uosm	Urinary osmolality
USG	Ultrasound
VAP	Ventilator-associated pneumonia
VAS	Visual analog score
VC	Vital capacity or volume control
VF	Ventricular fibrillation
VP	Venous pressure

VRSA	Vancomycin-resistant *Staphylococcus aureus*
VT	Ventricular tachycardia
V_T	Tidal volume
WBCs	White blood cells

EU GSPR Authorised Reprsentative
Logos Europe, 9 rue Nicolas Poussin
1700, La Rochelle, France
Phone: +33 (0) 6 67 93 73 78
E-mail: contact@logoseurope.eu

www.ingramcontent.com/pod-product-compliance
Ingram Content Group UK Ltd.
Pitfield, Milton Keynes, MK11 3LW, UK
UKHW041655270226
468476UK00007B/70